THE
EVERYTHING®

SMART
NUTRITION

MINI BOOK

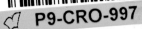
P9-CRO-997

Barbara Ravage

Adams Media Corporation
Avon, Massachusetts

Copyright ©2002, Adams Media Corporation.
All rights reserved. This book, or parts thereof, may not be
reproduced in any form without permission from the publisher;
exceptions are made for brief excerpts used in published reviews.

An Everything® Series Book.
"Everything" is a registered trademark of Adams Media Corporation.

Published by Adams Media Corporation
57 Littlefield Street, Avon, MA 02322
www.adamsmedia.com

ISBN: 1-58062-606-8

Printed in Canada.

J I H G F E D C B A

Library of Congress Cataloging-in-Publication Data
available from the publisher.

This publication is designed to provide accurate and authoritative information with regard to the subject matter covered. It is sold with the understanding that the publisher is not engaged in rendering legal, accounting, or
other professional advice. If legal advice or other expert assistance is
required, the services of a competent professional person should be sought.
— From a *Declaration of Principles* jointly adopted by a Committee of the
American Bar Association and a Committee of Publishers and Associations

Cover illustrations by Barry Littmann.
Interior illustrations by Barry Littmann.
Additional contributions by Susan Gaber.

This book is available at quantity discounts for bulk purchases.
For information, call 1-800-872-5627.

Contents

Introduction

If the last time you learned about food and nutrition was when you were in grade school, you may think it's "kid stuff." In fact, being smart about nutrition can be a matter of life and death. Many serious diseases and health conditions are caused by poor nutrition, and many others are made worse by it. Diabetes, high blood pressure, and heart disease are the biggies. Many cancers are thought to be more common in people who eat an unhealthful diet. And I'm not talking about malnutrition of the

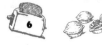

sort seen in poor and developing countries. I am talking about the way people eat in the wealthiest nation in the world.

In a sense, though, smart nutrition *is* kid stuff. But it's also teen stuff, adult stuff, middle-age stuff, and golden years stuff. It is vitally important no matter how old you are.

- Children need it as their brains and bodies grow and develop.
- Teens need it as their hormones play a larger role in their maturing bodies and they develop greater muscle and bone mass.
- Women need it when they are pregnant or nursing babies, but also throughout their lives, as protection against the loss of bone density that signals osteoporosis.

- Men need it to make hormones and to build and maintain their greater bone and muscle mass.
- Adults of both sexes need it to protect against cardiovascular disease and other serious health problems related to being overweight and underactive.
- Older people need it to maintain their health, strength, and vitality.
- We all need it to keep our bodies running, our brains working, and our immune systems on the alert.

When most people think about nutrition, they're thinking about dieting to lose weight. Too often that means *unbalancing* their

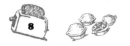

diet in an effort to eat less. Some weight-loss diets are designed to be unbalanced. Extreme low-calorie diets, eat-all-the-fat-you want diets, fasts, single-food regimens, and other quick weight-loss schemes are only a few of these. Others just end up being unbalanced as the frustrated dieter gives in to cravings after a period of deprivation.

Weight loss happens when you consume fewer calories than your body needs to do its work; weight gain happens when you consume more calories than your body needs, so the excess is stored as fat. Dieting is largely a matter of counting calories, but not all calories are equal.

Fat has twice as many calories, by weight, as do proteins and carbohydrates, the other two major nutrients. That makes a high-fat diet "expensive" from the point of view of calories, as well as risky from the point of view of health. Obesity, high cholesterol, high blood pressure, and other heart problems are much more common in people who eat a high-fat diet. Diabetes, the number one crippler in our nation today, is directly tied to dietary fat and obesity.

In the pages that follow, I'll be talking a lot about dietary fat—the kind that's found in the food we eat. Reducing the amount of fat you eat on a daily basis is one of the cornerstones of smart nutrition, and it's easier to do it than you may think.

Eating smart is a good way to lose weight, but it is also a good way to gain (if that's what you want to do) or maintain. It will provide you with the energy you need to lead an active, healthy lifestyle; it will keep your muscles, organs, and other body parts in good working order; it will strengthen your immune system, help you sleep well, and brighten your mood. Learning to be a smart eater is the best thing you can do for yourself and your loved ones. In fact, it's probably the most important lesson since you were back in grade school.

So, here's to smart nutrition, and to your health!

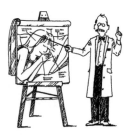

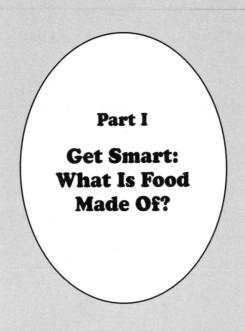

Part I

Get Smart: What Is Food Made Of?

What Is a Calorie?

You're probably used to thinking about calories as something found in the food you eat. Some foods are high in calories, others are low. In fact, a calorie is a measurement of energy. Technically speaking, though, a calorie is a unit of heat energy. It is equal to the amount of energy needed to raise the temperature of one cubic centimeter of water by one degree centigrade.

Calories in Food

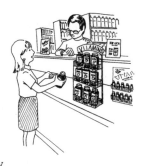

The caloric content of food is determined by burning a representative sample in a closed chamber in a laboratory. The amount of heat given off is measured, and that tells the lab technician how many calories were in that amount of food. The calorie values you find in calorie counters, diet books, and on the labels of the foods you buy are all based on this kind of lab work.

The U.S. Department of Agriculture (USDA) keeps track of this information in a huge database. If you have access to the Internet and want to look up the calorie content of any food you can imagine, *www.nal.usda.gov/fnic/cgi-bin/nut_search.pl* will

get you to the USDA Nutrient Database for
Standard Reference.

Calories in Your Body

Every time you eat something, you are taking in
energy that you can spend or save. You spend it
when you engage in physical activity, whether it
is blinking your eyes or running a marathon.
Your body also spends it for normal functions
such as breathing, moving blood through your
blood vessels, maintaining your body temperature
at 98.6 degrees Fahrenheit, building bone and
muscle tissue, and all the other tasks that keep
you alive from day to day.

Any energy left over is stored by your body
for future use. It doesn't matter whether what
you ate was fat or protein or carbohydrate, the

body stores excess energy in fat cells. Too many grapes turn into fat just as too much bacon does. As a general rule, 3,500 calories equals 1 pound of stored fat.

That's why we say people who eat more than they need are fat. They have more fat cells than people who are of normal weight. An adult whose weight is normal has about 30 billion fat cells. A person who is overweight might have more than three times as many, or 100 billion. People who are severely obese can have as many as 270 billion fat cells!

Unfortunately, once the body has made a fat cell, it's there forever. It may have less fat stored in it, but it sticks around waiting to be filled whenever the person takes in more calories than are needed. So even when a person loses weight, the number of fat cells does not

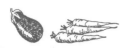

decrease. In fact, if all the existing fat cells are full, the body simply makes more. That's a very good reason to eat sensibly and stay active so your weight is within the normal range throughout your life.

Humans get their energy from food. (Plants get it from sunlight, which is another form of energy, of course.) When food is digested, it is processed by the body and broken down so it can be either used or stored. This is called metabolism, a term that refers to all the chemical processes involved in digesting and converting food into forms that can be used or stored in the body.

We are able to do this with three basic kinds of nutrients: fat, carbohydrate, and protein. You'll be learning more about those nutrients in the next few chapters. For now, all you have to remember is that calories are energy, whether they are going into your body as food or going out of it as activity.

How Many Calories Do You Need?

The number of calories an individual needs to maintain all body processes differs according to many variables. A person's age, his or her activity level, gender, and current weight all influence how many calories are needed. The rate of metabolism also influences how calories are burned and stored in the body. Figuring out how much you need to keep your weight the same, or to lose or gain weight, involves some complicated calculations. Some general guidelines for maintaining weight (neither gaining nor losing) have been set however. Use the following table to see how many calories a person of your age, weight, and gender needs every day to stay the same weight.

Recommended Calorie Intake

(by age, gender, and weight)

Age	Weight in pounds	Daily calorie intake
Infants		
to 6 months	13	650
6–12 months	20	850
Children		
1–3 years	29	1300
4–6 years	44	1800
7–10 years	52	2000
Teens, Female		
11–14 years	101	2200
15–18 years	120	2200

Recommended Calorie Intake
(continued)
(by age, gender, and weight)

Age	Weight in pounds	Daily calorie intake
Teens, Male		
11–14 years	99	2500
15–18 years	145	3000
Adults, Female		
19–24 years	128	2200
25–50 years	138	2200
51+ years	143	1900
Pregnant: add 300 calories/day for second and third trimester		
Lactating: add 500 calories/day		
Adults, Male		
19–24 years	160	2900
25–50 years	174	2900
51+ years	170	2300

These are approximate figures only. If you want to figure out how many calories a person of your age, gender, height, weight, and activity levels needs, numerous weight-loss and nutrition sites on the Internet feature calculators for this purpose.

Losing weight, of course, is a more complicated matter. Theoretically, you can do this by reducing your calorie intake over a period of time at the rate of 3,500 calories per pound you wish to lose. It will be far more effective, realistic, and lasting to reduce calorie intake *and* increase your level of activity. You will not only lose weight; you will also look and feel better, and improve your overall health.

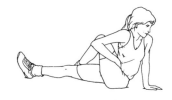

Chapter 2

What Are Fats?

Fats are the first of the three major nutrient groups you'll be learning about. It's important to know, however, that even though I'll be talking about each group separately, most of the food we eat contains a combination of the three. It is rare to find a food that is pure protein or pure carbohydrate. Fat is an exception. Oils, whether they are olive oil or coconut oil, fish oil or sunflower oil, or anything in between, are pure fat. So are butter, suet, and lard.

But what is a fat? Members of a family of chemical compounds called lipids, fats are molecules that cannot be dissolved in water. They are found in many plants and animals, which use them as storehouses of energy just as humans do.

How Much Fat Do You Need?

The ideal daily amount of fat a person eats is a matter of debate. The American Heart Association and federal government health agencies, for example, recommend that no more than 30 percent of a person's daily calories should come from fat. Other experts think 20 percent is a healthier figure, and yet others would lower it to 10 percent. Researchers are studying the impact on health of various levels, and it is hoped

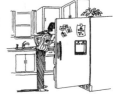

that a more definite recommendation will come out of those studies. If you are like most Americans, however, chances are that your daily diet contains more fat than you need.

A diet that is totally free from fat would be an unhealthy one indeed. Although it is true that carbohydrates provide storable energy, that is short-term storage at best. The body can store no more than 12 hours' worth of energy from carbohydrates, whereas an adult of average weight normally stores enough fat to keep the body running for two months! Fat is the most compact supply of food energy, more than twice that of carbohydrates and protein. In times of famine, that's a big plus. In times of plenty, it can be a big problem.

In the food we eat, fat is the major carrier of flavor. It's a simple fact, though perhaps an unfortunate one, that fat is a big part of what makes food taste good. Fat also does a better job of making us feel satisfied by what we've eaten than protein and carbohydrates do. The feeling of fullness, or satiety, comes mostly from fat.

Before considering the kind of fat you eat, let's take a look at the fat in your body, and especially the fat in your blood.

Fat in Your Body

Aside from energy storage, fats play many important roles in the human body. When they are released from storage they can be used for energy. They carry nutrients to many cells. They transport the fat-soluble vitamins A, D, E, and K. They keep our skin supple and our hair shiny.

They provide insulation and are used to make hormones and elements of the immune system. They cushion our organs and form the membrane of all the cells in our bodies. They are an important constituent of the nervous system. They are a source of fatty acids, which are used for normal growth and development. But for all its benefits, fat has an ugly side, and I'm not just talking about the way it looks on your hips and around your waist.

Study after study has shown that a diet high in fat leads to high levels of cholesterol in the blood, which contributes to clogging of the arteries (atherosclerosis), which in turn may result in high blood pressure, heart disease, heart attack, and stroke. Diabetes and certain cancers have also been connected to diets high in fat.

What Is Cholesterol?

In addition to the fat stored in cells, there are fat-like chemicals in the lipid family circulating in your blood. The most infamous of these is cholesterol, a waxy substance the body uses to make cell membranes and brain and nerve tissue. It is also needed for the production of steroid hormones and acids used in digestion. Cholesterol is not, in and of itself, a bad thing. Too much cholesterol of the wrong type can be harmful to your health, however.

Cholesterol can get into your body through food, but your body actually makes all the cholesterol it needs. The liver is the cholesterol factory. The bloodstream is the highway cholesterol uses to get where it needs to go, and the vehicle cholesterol travels in is a combination fat-protein molecule called a lipoprotein.

There are several different types of lipoprotein; the two important ones are low-density and high-density. Cholesterol carried in low-density lipoproteins is called LDL cholesterol. The kind carried in high-density lipoproteins is called HDL cholesterol. I am sure you have heard these terms, and probably also know that LDL cholesterol is considered the "bad" cholesterol and HDL the "good" one.

How can cholesterol be both good and bad? The answer lies in the different ways the two types act in your body. LDL cholesterol promotes formation of fatty deposits, called plaques, on the inner walls of the arteries, causing them to narrow. Not only does this decrease the amount of blood flowing through the arteries, it also increases the pressure needed to push the blood along. In addition, the rough inner walls promote the formation of blood clots, which can cause strokes, heart attacks, and other serious health problems. Not only does HDL not do this, it seems to inhibit plaque formation, working against LDL.

What all this means is that it's a good idea to have a lower level of LDL and a higher level of HDL in your blood. In fact, that's a good way to remember this rule: L for "low" and LDL; H for "high" and HDL.

There is another type of lipid that has an effect on health. This is called triglyceride, and it is carried through the blood in very low-density lipoproteins, or VLDL. As you might imagine, if LDL is bad, VLDL is very bad. High levels of triglycerides go hand in hand with high LDL and low HDL. People with diabetes or kidney disease often have high triglyceride levels. Your doctor may also have your blood tested for triglycerides, especially if you have higher than normal cholesterol levels or other health problems caused by this.

New Cholesterol Guidelines

When it comes to cholesterol (and triglycerides), what is low and what is high?

In 2001, the National Heart, Lung, and Blood Institute, a division of the National Institutes of Health, issued new guidelines on cholesterol. They are the result of studies showing how harmful high LDL cholesterol levels can be and how great the benefits of lowering those levels are. They not only set new limits for what is considered an optimal (or healthy) level of LDL, but they also urge doctors to be more aggressive in working with their patients to lower their LDL.

Strategies include a low-fat diet, exercise, and, if necessary, cholesterol-lowering drugs.

The new guidelines deal with total cholesterol (the sum of LDL and HDL), as well as the two types separately and triglycerides. Lowering LDL cholesterol is considered the primary target. For that reason, the characterization "near or above optimal" refers to two situations: "near" means a person who is trying to lower LDL is close to being successful; "above" means that a person who is not being treated for high cholesterol should reduce fat in his or her diet, increase activity, and possibly take cholesterol-lowering drugs.

The New Guidelines

Total Cholesterol (mg/dL)	Level
less than 200	desirable
200–239	borderline high
240 or more	high

LDL Cholesterol (mg/dL)	Level
less than 100	optimal
100–129	near or above optimal
130–159	borderline high
160–189	high
190 or more	very high

HDL Cholesterol (mg/dL)	Level
less than 40	low
60 or more	high

Triglycerides (mg/dL)	Level
less than 150	normal
150–199	borderline high
200–499	high
500 or more	very high

When you have your blood tested for cholesterol, you will get a figure for "total cholesterol," the combination of LDL and HDL, expressed as milligrams per deciliter (mg/dL). That means how many milligrams (1/1000 of a gram) of cholesterol there are in each deciliter ($^1/_{10}$ of a liter) of your blood. The new guidelines recommend that all healthy adults have a complete lipoprotein profile done every five years. People with a variety of health problems (a previous high cholesterol result, diabetes, obesity, heart disease, and high blood pressure, among them) should have it done more often.

A complete lipoprotein profile includes measures of total cholesterol, LDL, HDL, and triglycerides. The most accurate test is done after you have not eaten for nine to 12 hours.

Fighting High Cholesterol

High cholesterol and triglyceride levels can be treated with medicine, and in the past decade some new and very effective drugs have been invented for this purpose. Changing eating habits can also significantly lower cholesterol levels for most people. Exceptions include those whose high cholesterol levels are related to certain genetic characteristics. Even when a person takes cholesterol-lowering medication, however, doctors recommend changing the diet to one that is low in fat.

This is a good idea for everyone, whether high cholesterol is currently a problem or not.

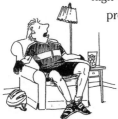

The Fats You Eat

There are three main types of fats (or fatty acids, to get technical about it): saturated, monounsaturated, and polyunsaturated. These terms refer to the number of paired hydrogen atoms that are linked with the carbon atoms that make up a fat molecule. Without sending us back to high-school chemistry class, let's just say that saturated fats have as many hydrogen atoms as there are available notches—they are fully saturated with hydrogen—whereas monounsaturated fats have room for one additional pair and polyunsaturated fats have room for more than one additional pair.

Here's a much easier way to remember the difference:

- Saturated fat is solid at room temperature: butter, lard, and tallow are saturated fats.

- Monounsaturated fat is liquid at room temperature and begins to thicken (or get cloudy) when it is refrigerated: olive, peanut, and canola oils are monounsaturated fats.

- Polyunsaturated fat is liquid at both room temperature and under refrigeration; it does not thicken or get cloudy when it is chilled: safflower, corn, and blended vegetable oils are polyunsaturated fats.

Good Guys and Bad Guys

If that's the difference, what difference does it make? All fats, no matter what kind, contain nine calories per gram, so if you're watching calories, it makes no difference. On the other hand, unsaturated fats do not promote artery clogging, whereas saturated fats do, so if you're concerned about the effect on heart and circulatory health, it makes a big difference.

Another big difference has to do with your blood cholesterol level. You can't choose foods by whether they have HDL or LDL. On the way into your body, cholesterol in food is just cholesterol. The difference comes through what your body does with it. For complicated reasons that are not fully understood, saturated fats tend to raise levels of LDL. Polyunsaturated fats lower levels of both LDL and HDL, whereas monounsaturated fats lower levels of LDL but do not affect HDL levels. That makes saturated fats the bad guys and unsaturated fats the good guys, with monounsaturated fats the better of the good guys.

When choosing fats to eat, the best approach is to:

- Limit saturated fats. Most experts advise that less than 10 percent of total caloric intake should come from saturated fat.

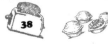

- Get most of your dietary fat from unsaturated sources. Total fat intake should not exceed 30 percent of your daily calories.
- Choose olive, peanut, and canola oil more often than safflower, corn, and other vegetable oils.

Exceptions to the Rule

In general, fats from animal sources (meat and poultry, as well as eggs, cheese, and other dairy products) contain saturated fat. Plant and vegetable oils (including nut oils) are sources of unsaturated fats. Three exceptions are palm, palm kernel, and coconut oils. Even though these are from plant sources, the fat they contain is saturated. It is advisable, though not always easy, to avoid these fats.

The reason why it isn't easy can be found on the label of many baked goods. Because of their good flavor and ability to stay fresh longer, one or more of these oils are commonly used in crackers, cakes, and other bakery items. If you do your own baking from scratch, you can control this, but store-bought baked goods and cake mixes are a notorious source of these three "exceptional" oils.

Some Other Good Guys: Omega Oils

The term omega refers to the molecular structure of certain polyunsaturated fat molecules. There are two important types: omega-3 and omega-6. They contribute to normal nervous system development and play an important part in metabolism and hormone activity. Recent research suggests they may

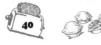

protect against health problems ranging from rheumatoid arthritis and lupus to cancer, high blood pressure, and heart disease. Omega-3s lower the level of triglycerides in the blood and also reduce the likelihood of blood clots. Although still unproven, some researchers believe they can also decrease the severity of childhood asthma.

The omegas are considered essential fatty acids. That is, the body needs them but cannot make them, so we must rely on food to provide us with enough.

How much is enough? Knowledge about omega oils is still incomplete, and there are no daily recommendations for them. For the present, experts think as little as two servings of fatty fish per week will provide what the average person needs. Still, it is believed that most

Americans get only one tenth of the omegas that they should.

Omega-3s are found in fish, particularly fatty fish like salmon and mackerel. Shellfish, sardines, tuna, mullet, herring, trout, and anchovies are other good fish sources. They are also found in nuts (especially walnuts), flaxseed, wheat germ, soybeans, and soy and canola oils. Dark green leafy vegetables (spinach and kale, for example) are another source. The best source for babies is breast milk, which is rich in omega-3.

Soybean oil is also a source of omega-6 fatty acids, as are corn and safflower oils. Egg yolks, organ meats, and other animal products are other good sources.

Fish oil capsules and other supplements can provide omega-3, but most nutritional experts agree that foods are the best way to get these essential nutrients. In Chapter 5 I'll be talking more about the role of micronutrients in a smart diet, and will discuss the pros and cons of supplements.

Two Good News/Bad News Fats

There's another lipid that promises the taste benefits of fat without the health risks. This "designer fat" is called Olestra. It's a synthetic fat that is not absorbed by the body. For that reason, it supplies no calories and never gets into your blood or stored in your fat cells. You cannot buy it to cook with or spread on bread, but it has been approved by the federal Food and Drug Administration (FDA) for use in certain snack foods, most notably potato chips.

The problem is that eating a lot of Olestra-fried food results in some extremely unpleasant digestive sensations. I'll spare you the details. It is also thought that it interferes with the way your body gets its fat-soluble vitamins. For these reasons, Olestra is not a useful universal fat substitute.

Benecol is another designer fat. It is absorbed by your body, and therefore supplies the same nine calories per gram as any other fat. Its benefit is that it appears to be able to lower cholesterol levels. It can be bought in margarine, cheese, and a few other foods. The cholesterol-lowering effect lasts only as long as you continue eating it, however, which makes it almost like medicine. Some medical experts think it should be regulated by the FDA, just as drugs are, and there is a possibility this may happen in the future. Until then, it's not a bad idea to talk to your doctor about using it if you are concerned about your cholesterol level.

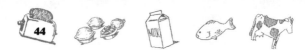

The Ultimate Bad Guys: Trans Fats

Trans fatty acids are polyunsaturated fats that have been "engineered" to act like saturated fats. That is, they are solid at room temperature, they have the "mouth-feel" of saturated fats like butter, and they are less likely to become rancid, so the foods they are prepared with stay fresher longer. Sounds great, doesn't it? So good, in fact, that solid (stick) margarine relies on them to make it a convincing butter substitute and they are used in many baked goods to give them a longer shelf life.

The process of making trans fats is called hydrogenation, because it involves adding hydrogen atoms to unsaturated fats, saturating them. This process not only makes them act like

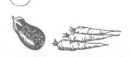

saturated fat in food, it makes them act like saturated fat in your body.

- They raise the level of cholesterol in your blood, especially LDL, the "bad" cholesterol.
- They raise the level of triglycerides in your blood.
- They contribute to cardiovascular disease, including atherosclerosis and high blood pressure, heart attack, and stroke.

The bottom line, it should be clear, is that trans fats should be avoided whenever possible. But that's easier said than done.

Trans fats are sometimes called "stealth fats." That's because current food labeling regulations do not require that they be listed separately

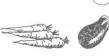

on food labels. The law may change, but until it does:

- Choose liquid, squeezable margarine rather than the solid, stick kind.
- Read food labels and limit or avoid altogether foods containing "hydrogenated" or "partially hydrogenated" fats and oils.

So, now you have the skinny on fats. In Chapter 9, I'll talk about what you can do to reduce the amount of fat in your diet.

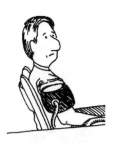

What Are Proteins?

The second major nutrient group you'll be learning about are proteins. Like fats, these are acid molecules, amino acids to be specific. Often called the body's building blocks, amino acids are used to make many different kinds of cells. Your skin, hair, nails, bones, muscles, and organs are all made from amino acids. So are your genes. Hormones, digestive enzymes, and immune system cells also owe their existence to amino acids. Your body uses amino acids to repair

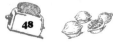

damaged cells and to make new ones, especially during the growing years but also throughout the life span. In fact, without proteins, life itself would be impossible.

There are 80 amino acids found in nature, but humans need only 20 to keep their bodies running. The body can make some of the 20, but others have to be obtained from foods. Those we need to get from food are called essential amino acids.

Proteins also supply energy to the body, at the rate of four calories per gram, a bit less than half the amount supplied by fat. They are not as readily available a source of energy as carbohydrates and fat are, however, because it is more complicated to break them down and it takes more energy to do so. Under famine conditions, the body first uses stored fat to provide energy, and only when fat stores are used up does it start drawing on muscles, the body's own protein bank. It is rare to see muscle wasting because of malnutrition in the developed world, though it is, sadly, a common sight in countries where food is scarce.

How Much Protein Do You Need?

The average adult needs about half a gram of protein for every pound of body weight. People who have very muscular bodies need more, as do people who are ill and women who are pregnant or breastfeeding their babies. But the real protein hogs are babies and children. Because their bodies are growing rapidly, they need a lot of amino acid building blocks, infants about three times and children and teens about twice as much, *per pound of body weight*, as adults.

A good rule of thumb is that 10 percent of your daily intake of calories should come from protein. So, for example, if you should be eating 2,000 calories each day, 200 of them should be from protein. At four calories per gram, your daily protein intake should be 50 grams of protein.

Based on average weights, the following chart shows roughly what the daily protein intake should be. Keep in mind that your weight may not be average. Other factors that influence protein needs are the ratio of muscle to bone and fat in your body, how active you are, and the general state of your health.

Protein Needs

Age	Recommended daily protein intake (grams)
Children	
birth–6 months	13
7–12 months	14
1–3 years	16
4–6 years	24
7–10 years	28
Males	
11–14	45
15–18	59
19–24	58
25+	63
Females	
11–14	46
15–18	44
19–24	46
25+	50
Pregnant	60
Lactating	62–65

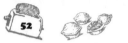

Food Sources of Protein

The richest sources of protein in the food we eat come from animals, including fish. Milk, cheese, and eggs are all animal products, and good sources of protein. People who do not eat animal products, however, can still get the protein they need. Nuts, beans, and other vegetables contain proteins, though in smaller quantities.

The reason why animal sources are considered the best way to get protein is because they provide what are called "complete" proteins. That is, they contain all the essential amino acids. Many vegetables contain some but not all of them. This can be solved by careful combining of vegetables. For example, the classic combination of rice and beans will give you all the essential amino acids in the correct proportions. That's probably why it is a staple dish in many of the world's cuisines.

People who follow a vegetarian diet do need to be more careful about getting enough protein to keep their bodies healthy. In Chapter 10, you will find a listing for a Web site called the Vegetarian Resource Group, which provides valuable information and links for people who choose a vegetarian way of eating.

Protein's Fellow Travelers

Earlier in this book I said that it is rare to find a food that is made of only one nutrient type. This is especially true of proteins, and even more true of proteins from animal sources. Animal protein tends to be accompanied by animal fat, which as you now know is saturated fat. Four ounces of steak may look like a big hunk of protein to you, but

it is surrounded by and permeated with fat.
The same goes for cheese and eggs, both
major sources of saturated fat.

That is one of the reasons why some
people prefer to get more of their protein from
vegetables, which are a major source of carbohydrates and a lesser source of protein.

Read on to learn about carbohydrates, the
third nutrient group.

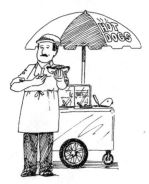

What Are Carbohydrates?

For reasons that mystify me, carbohydrates have recently gotten a bad name, with talk about carbohydrate addiction and promotion of high-fat/low-carb weight-loss diets. In fact, carbohydrates are the foundation of healthful eating.

They are your body's principal source of energy, the easiest of the nutrients for your body to turn into fuel or to store for future needs. Furthermore, they are truly "brain food," since your brain cannot use either of the other two nutrients to keep it humming.

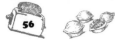

Like proteins, each gram of carbohydrate supplies the body with four calories. And like fats and proteins, carbohydrates are molecules, but they can be simple or complex ones. Most carbohydrate foods contain a combination of simple and complex types:

- Sugars are simple carbohydrates. In food, they may take the form of sucrose (table sugar), lactose, fructose, dextrose, or maltose. It's pretty obvious that sugar is found in fruits (fructose), but even foods that do not taste sweet—milk and many vegetables, for example—contain simple sugars.
- Starches are complex carbohydrates. Grains and grain products (bread, pasta, and breakfast cereal, for instance) are major sources of complex carbohydrates. Other

sources include fruits, vegetables, beans, and some dairy products.

- Fiber, or cellulose, is a very complex carbohydrate. What this means is that the molecule is constructed in such a complicated way that the human body cannot digest it at all. That makes it an extremely interesting dietary component.

There are two types of fiber:

- Soluble fiber can be dissolved in water; dried beans, oats, barley, apples, citrus, and vegetables are sources of soluble fiber.
- Insoluble fiber does not dissolve in water; wheat bran, whole grains, cereals, seeds, and fruit and vegetable skins are sources of insoluble fiber.

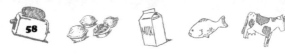

How Much Carbohydrate Do You Need?

If you've been keeping track of the recommended percent of daily calorie intake I've told you about so far (no more than 30 percent fat and 10 percent protein), you will not be surprised to hear that 60 percent of your daily calories should come from carbohydrates. And if you've ever taken a look at the Food Guide Pyramid, you now know why carbohydrates form the wide base of that triangular chart.

If you should eat 3,000 calories a day to maintain a healthy weight, no fewer than 1,800 of them should come from carbohydrates. If your intake should be 2,000 calories, carbohydrates should add up to 1,200 of them.

But there is a catch. Well, really, there are two.

Complex Is Better Than Simple

Simple carbohydrates, or sugars, go right into your blood. They may provide a quick burst of energy, but they do not last. Nutritionally, they don't do much for you, which is why they are sometimes called "empty" calories. Complex carbohydrates, on the other hand, can be used or stored for the future. Furthermore, your body works pretty hard at processing them, burning calories as it performs that task. That makes them a pretty good "diet food." They tend to be bulky, which makes you feel full after you have eaten them. Unlike protein foods, complex carbohydrates often travel without fat or with low levels of it, and that fat is almost always the unsaturated kind. And carbohydrate-rich foods are also rich in vitamins and minerals.

Current dietary guidelines urge emphasizing complex carbohydrates. Between grains, fruits,

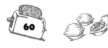

and vegetables, you should eat a total of eleven to twenty servings of carbohydrate-containing foods each day.

Fiber Is Your Friend

The other catch has to do with fiber. You might think that fiber is useless if your body cannot use it. In fact, fiber provides no calories but it provides many valuable services:

- It adds bulk to the diet, giving you a feeling of fullness that lasts quite a while after you finish eating. Lettuce and other salad vegetables, for example, are mostly fiber and water. A bowl of salad will do more to make you feel full than an amount of meat that is equal in calories.

- Soluble fiber lowers blood cholesterol levels, reducing the risk of heart disease.

- Fiber appears to lower the risk of developing diabetes.
- It passes through the stomach and into the intestines without losing bulk, which helps maintain bowel regularity and avoid constipation.
- Insoluble fiber acts as an intestinal cleanser, especially by reducing the likelihood of diverticulitis, a very painful inflammation that results when small pouches in the inner walls of the intestines get clogged with feces.
- Fiber may guard against some cancers, especially cancer of the colon. The way it does this is not known for sure, but it has been observed that people who eat plenty of fiber are less likely to develop

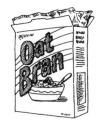

colon cancer than people whose diet is fiber poor.

In view of all that, it makes sense to eat enough fiber every day. Most people get only about 10 grams of fiber in their daily diet, when between 20 and 30 grams is recommended. Eating more than that may cause digestive discomfort, without adding much in the way of benefits.

Where's the Fiber?

Fiber is found only in plant foods. Following are some good sources of fiber:

- whole grains, especially oats, oat and wheat bran, and barley
- dried beans
- nuts

- dried fruits, such as raisins, prunes, dates, and figs
- fresh fruits, especially pears, apples, and citrus
- edible seeds, including sunflower and sesame
- vegetables, including potatoes, carrots, and celery
- fruit and vegetable skins

I hope you no longer think of carbohydrates as something to be avoided. Smart nutrition means eating a balanced diet. Building that diet on the sturdy foundation of complex carbohydrates is one of the smartest things you can do.

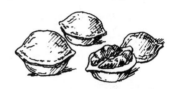

5 What Are Micronutrients?

Aside from fat, protein, and carbohydrates, food contains chemicals that exist in tiny amounts but have benefits that far exceed their weight. These are the micronutrients—vitamins and minerals.

Instead of measuring them in grams, ounces, or even pounds, they are measured in milligrams (thousandths of a gram, abbreviated "mg") and micrograms (millionths of a gram, abbreviated "mcg")!

They may be small, but there are a lot of them, and they do a lot for you. I'll tell you a bit about vitamins and minerals in this chapter, but if you want to know more than can fit in this small book, *The Everything® Vitamins, Minerals, and Nutritional Supplements Book* and *The Everything® Vitamins Mini Book*, both by Maureen Ternus, M.S., R.D., and Kitty Broihier, M.S., R.D. (Adams Media), are excellent sources of comprehensive information.

Vitamins

Vitamins are complex organic molecules that, in general, cannot be made by the body and must, therefore, be obtained from food sources. There are three exceptions to this rule: vitamin A, which the body makes from carotene; vitamin D, which is formed when ultraviolet light is absorbed by our skin; and vitamin K, which is made by friendly bacteria that live in our intestines.

Vitamins contain no calories and thus are not a source of energy. Our bodies use them to make, maintain, and repair cells. They also play a big part in metabolism, which means we could not absorb, process, store, and use food without them.

Vitamins are generally classified as water- or fat-soluble. The water-soluble vitamins are the B complex (thiamin, riboflavin, niacin, pantothenic acid, pyridoxine, biotin, folate, and cobalamin) and C. They are taken in with food and used or eliminated through urine. They cannot be stored and so should be part of everyday eating.

The fat-soluble vitamins are A, D, E, and K. They are found in foods containing fat and can be stored in fat cells of the body. These two facts make fat-soluble vitamins a more complicated matter than water-soluble ones. On the one hand, consuming more than the body needs (by taking large doses of vitamin supplements, for example) can result over time in a build-up of toxic levels of these vitamins, something that does not happen with water-soluble ones, since the excess is flushed away. On the other hand, very low-fat diets or medical conditions that interfere with fat digestion can result in deficiencies of these vitamins.

About Antioxidants

Some vitamins have antioxidant properties, which makes them especially important in maintaining health. A number of health problems are associated with cell damage caused

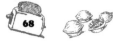

by free radicals, which can be thought of as "rogue" oxygen molecules released as byproducts of metabolism. Free radicals also get into our bodies through exposure to environmental pollution and radiation from the sun and X-rays.

Free radicals have been linked to everything from cancer and cataracts to diabetes, stroke, and heart disease. Antioxidants, as the name suggests, help defend against oxidation damage from free radicals and thus may offer some protection against these diseases.

An important antioxidant is beta-carotene. This orange pigment is a "precursor" of vitamin A. That means it is used by the body to make vitamin A. Beta-carotene can be found in bright yellow and orange foods such as sweet potatoes and carrots, as well as in green leafy vegetables.

Following is a brief rundown of the vitamins that are important for good nutrition and health. It tells what each one does, what the best (mostly food) sources are, how much you need each day, and what might happen if you get either too much or too little. It is important to know, however, that a balanced diet will provide adequate amounts of vitamins, and that deficiencies are rare in people who follow smart nutrition strategies. Getting too much from food is unlikely, though it might happen if you take what are termed "megadoses" of vitamin supplements.

In general, children need smaller amounts of vitamins and minerals than adults and can be harmed by getting too much. For that reason, do not give children vitamin and mineral supplements unless a pediatrician tells you to.

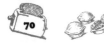

I'll talk more about supplements at the end of this chapter.

The Fat-Soluble Vitamins
Vitamin A (beta-carotene, retinol, retinal, retinoic acid)

What does it do? Helps develop and maintain normal vision, repair tissues, form bones; it is also important for reproduction, growth, hormone production, and skin and immune system health; beta-carotene acts as an antioxidant.

Where can you get it? Liver, orange vegetables (carrots, sweet potatoes), fortified foods (mostly dairy), eggs, oranges, green leafy vegetables, red fruits and vegetables.

How much do you need each day? 900 mcg for men, 700 mcg for women (between 1,200–1,300 mcg if they are breastfeeding);

children need between 375 mcg (for newborns) and 600 mcg by age 13.

Too much may lead to abdominal cramps, nausea, vomiting, diarrhea, loss of appetite, blurred vision, nosebleeds, hair loss, dry skin and skin rashes, irritability, dizziness, headaches, poor coordination; in extreme cases, red blood cell damage, liver disease, high cholesterol levels, and nervous system problems; birth defects are more common when a woman takes too much supplementary vitamin A.

Not enough may lead to night blindness, dry eyes, rough skin, greater susceptibility to infections; impaired bone formation in children.

Vitamin D

What does it do? Helps the body process and use calcium and phosphorus; essential for

72

bone and tooth health; helps muscle contraction and nerve signaling.

Where can you get it? Fish (especially canned salmon and sardines eaten with bones), liver, eggs; fortified milk and dairy foods; produced by the action of sunlight on skin.

How much do you need each day? In addition to exposure to sunlight, 200 IU (equivalent to 5 mcg) for adults, 400 IU (10 mcg) after age 50, and 600 IU (15 mcg) after age 70; 300 IU (7.5 mcg) for newborns and 400 IU (10 mcg) for children.

Too much may lead to excess calcium in blood and calcium deposits on soft tissues, constipation, kidney stones, loss of appetite, irritability, nausea, vomiting, thirst, weakness; in extreme cases, mental retardation and impaired growth in children; extreme over-doses can be fatal.

Not enough may lead to rickets (including bowlegs and short stature) in children, osteomalacia (fragile and painful bones) in adults; joint pain, muscle twitching and cramps, osteoporosis, soft bones, and bone deformities.

Vitamin E

What does it do? Acts as an antioxidant; protects cell membranes, including red blood cells.

Where can you get it? Nuts, whole grains, wheat germ; green leafy vegetables; vegetable and seed oils.

How much do you need each day? 15 mg for adults, 19 mg for pregnant and breastfeeding women; 11 mg for preteens.

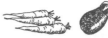

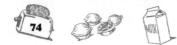

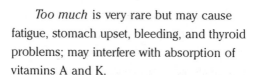

Too much is very rare but may cause fatigue, stomach upset, bleeding, and thyroid problems; may interfere with absorption of vitamins A and K.

Not enough is uncommon in healthy people, but occurs in those with diseases that interfere with fat absorption; may lead to anemia, bleeding, neurological and reproductive problems, and impaired immunity.

Vitamin K

What does it do? Active in blood clotting and regulation of calcium in blood; helps metabolism of protein.

Where can you get it? Seaweed, green tea, cabbage, brussels sprouts, spinach, broccoli, kale, and other leafy greens; it is also made by "friendly" bacteria in the intestines.

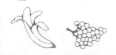

How much do you need each day? 120 mcg for men, 90 mcg for women, 60 mcg for teens; children need between 5 mcg (for newborns) and 30 mcg (by age 10).

Too much may lead to jaundice.

Not enough may lead to bleeding.

The Water-Soluble Vitamins
Vitamin C (ascorbic acid)

What does it do? Acts as an antioxidant; aids in absorption of iron, wound healing, production of collagen and hormones, and resistance to infection; and helps keep bones, blood vessels, and teeth healthy.

Where can you get it? Citrus, berries, kiwi fruit, melon, mangoes, papaya, tomatoes, potatoes, sweet and hot peppers, leafy green vegetables.

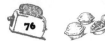

How much do you need each day? 90 mg for men, 75 mg for women, 85 mg during pregnancy and 120 mg while breastfeeding; children need between 15 mg beginning at age 3 and 45 mg by age 13.

Too much is rarely a problem but may lead to damage to red blood cells, blood in stools, and stress to diseased kidneys and liver.

Not enough may lead to anemia and scurvy (swollen and bleeding gums, loose teeth, bleeding, joint pain, poor wound healing, weakness, fatigue, and impaired resistance to infection).

Thiamin (B₁)

What does it do? Helps metabolism of carbohydrates and proteins; helps make DNA and keep nervous system and appetite normal.

Where can you get it? Meat (especially pork), legumes, whole grain breads and cereals, pasta, sunflower seeds, nuts, brewer's yeast.

How much do you need each day? 1.1 mg for adults, 1.4 mg during pregnancy, and 1.5 mg while breastfeeding; children need 0.5 mg and teens 0.9 mg.

Too much is rare, but may cause weakness, headaches, irritability, insomnia, and a rapid pulse.

Not enough is uncommon but may occur in people with kidney disease, the elderly, women pregnant with twins or more, chronic dieters and alcoholics, and "extreme" athletes; may lead to beriberi, impaired growth in children, irregular heartbeat, high blood pressure, muscle weakness, swelling and

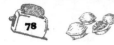

bloating, mental confusion and other nervous system problems.

Riboflavin (B₂)

What does it do? Helps metabolize carbo-hydrates, fats, and proteins.

Where can you get it? Milk and dairy prod-ucts, especially eggs and yogurt, liver, enriched breads and cereals.

How much do you need each day? 1.3 mg for men, 1.1 mg for women, 1.4 mg during preg-nancy, and 1.6 mg while breastfeeding; children need 0.5 mg.

Too much is rarely a problem.

Not enough may lead to vision and skin problems, weakness, sore throat, mouth sores, anemia, hypersensitivity to light.

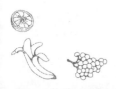

Niacin (vitamin B₃)

What does it do? Helps keep nerves, skin, and digestive system healthy, release stored energy, and regulate calcium use in body.

Where can you get it? Meat (especially liver), fish, eggs, poultry, cereals, legumes, nuts, seeds, milk, green leafy vegetables, brewer's yeast.

How much do you need each day? 16 mg for men; 14 mg for women, 18 mg during pregnancy and 17 mg while breastfeeding; teens need 12 mg.

Too much may cause low blood pressure, "niacin flush" (temporary tingling and reddening of the head and neck), headaches, nausea; in extreme cases, stomach ulcers and liver problems.

Not enough may lead to pellagra, skin rashes (especially on sun exposure), anemia, diarrhea, vomiting, loss of appetite, weakness, irritability,

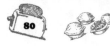

headache, and fatigue; in extreme cases, mental confusion, disorientation, and memory loss.

Pantothenic acid

What does it do? Helps metabolize carbohydrates and fats and make cholesterol, some hormones, and red blood cells.

Where can you get it? In many different foods, especially egg yolks, kidneys, liver, and brewer's yeast.

How much do you need each day? 5 mg for adults and teens, 6 mg during pregnancy and 7 mg while breastfeeding; children need between 2 mg (for newborns) to 4–7 mg by age 13.

Too much may cause diarrhea.

Not enough is rare, but may lead to nausea, fatigue, depression, insomnia, muscle weakness, numbness, and burning sensation in feet.

Pyridoxine (B_6)

What does it do? Helps metabolize fat and protein, produce blood sugar, and form red blood cells and antibodies.

Where can you get it? Meat, fish, bananas, green leafy vegetables, legumes, whole grains.

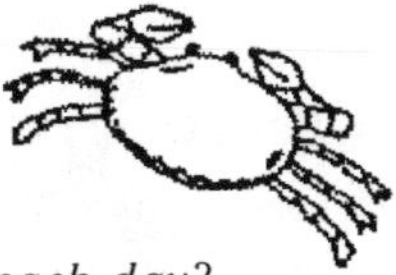

How much do you need each day? 1.3–1.7 mg for adults, 2 mg during pregnancy and breastfeeding; children need between 0.3 mg (for newborns) and 1.7 mg by age 14.

Too much may cause sensitivity to sunlight and nerve damage.

Not enough is rare, though the elderly and chronic alcoholics may be deficient; severe deficiency may lead to anemia, skin rashes, mouth sores and smooth tongue, kidney stones, muscle weakness, and seizures.

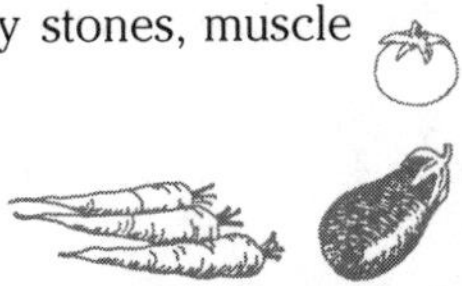

Biotin (vitamin H, coenzyme R)

What does it do? Helps metabolism, cell growth, and fetal development.

Where can you get it? In many different foods.

How much do you need each day? 30 mcg for adults, 35 mcg while breastfeeding; children need between 10 mcg (for newborns) and 25 mcg by age 18.

Too much is not a problem.

Not enough may lead to nausea and loss of appetite, thinning and loss of hair, depression, muscle pain and weakness, fatigue, skin rashes; in extreme cases, hallucinations.

Folate (folic acid, folacin)

What does it do? Helps make DNA; essential for cell division; takes part in making red blood cells and metabolism of proteins.

Where can you get it? Enriched breads, cereals, pasta, and rice; green leafy vegetables (especially asparagus, spinach, and other greens), legumes, liver, folate-fortified orange juice, seeds.

How much do you need each day? 400 mcg for adults; 600 mcg during pregnancy, and 500 mcg while breastfeeding; children need between 25 mcg (in infancy) and 300 mcg (by age 14).

Too much may mask B_{12} deficiency; may lead to diarrhea, insomnia, and irritability.

Not enough is quite common and may lead to anemia, weakness, fatigue, headache, irritability, shortness of breath, difficulty concentrating; severe birth defects may occur in children whose mothers do not get enough just before and in the earliest days of pregnancy.

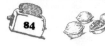

Cobalamin (B₁₂)

What does it do? Helps make red blood cells and keep the nervous system working.

Where can you get it? From animal products: meat, fish (especially shellfish), poultry, milk, eggs, cheese; also found in yeast.

How much do you need each day? 2 mcg for teens and adults; 2.6 mcg during pregnancy and breastfeeding; children need less (between 0.3 mcg for newborns and 1.4 mcg at age 10); vegetarians need to take supplements.

Too much is not a problem.

Not enough may lead to anemia, nerve damage, fatigue, depression; extreme deficiencies may lead to paralysis and mental confusion.

Minerals

Minerals are nonorganic elements or compounds that occur naturally in the soil and therefore are absorbed by living things—plants and animals— along with their food. Like vitamins, minerals exist in small amounts in what we eat and are necessary to our health. And like vitamins, they supply no calories, but perform important functions we could not live without, including helping transport oxygen to our cells, maintaining fluid balance throughout our bodies, manufacturing hormones, and keeping our heart beating and our blood pressure at normal levels. They play a part in forming our bones, our blood, and our digestive enzymes, and much more.

There are far more minerals of nutritional value than there are vitamins. In fact, there are too many and their functions are too complex to cover in this book. There are about eighty minerals present in the food we eat and in our bodies; of those 20 are considered essential. That is, they are necessary for human health and must be obtained from outside sources since the body cannot make them.

The essential minerals are divided in two categories. The major minerals are needed in amounts of 100 mg daily or more. They are:

- Calcium
- Chlorine
- Magnesium
- Phosphorus
- Potassium
- Sodium
- Sulfur

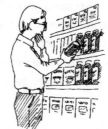

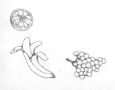

Thirteen other minerals are needed, but in smaller amounts, which is why they are called trace minerals. These are:

- Chromium
- Cobalt
- Copper
- Fluorine
- Iodine
- Iron
- Manganese
- Molybdenum
- Selenium
- Silicon
- Tin
- Vanadium
- Zinc

There are a few others that are probably essential, but little is known about the way they work. In general, you will get as much of the essential minerals as you need in a balanced diet, and will certainly do so if you take a single multivitamin/mineral supplement each day.

As with vitamins, it is important to get enough of each essential mineral but can be dangerous to ingest too much. In many cases, the excess is excreted with urine, but in others it is possible to build up toxic levels.

There are a few essential minerals worth singling out because of what happens when you do not get enough of them.

Calcium

We owe the hardness of our bones and teeth to calcium, the same mineral that is found in the shells of clams and oysters. Our bones form throughout childhood and begin "demineralizing" around age 35. This is part of the natural process of aging, but it can be a problem, for women

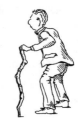

especially, if we live longer than our bones.
The greatest loss of bone mass occurs in the
years immediately preceding and following
menopause, due to the lower levels and even-
tual absence of the female hormone estrogen.
All women, therefore, need extra calcium, even
before they reach menopause and even if they
take estrogen replacement.

Milk and other dairy products are the
richest source of calcium, but many women do
not eat enough of those to get the amount they
need. Calcium supplements are a must for all
women, therefore.

The current recommendation for women is
1,300 mg from age nine to 18, 1,000 mg until age
50, and 1,200 mg thereafter. Some experts recommend as much as 1,500 mg after age 55 or the
onset of menopause. Because the body needs

vitamin D to use calcium effectively, adequate intake of that vitamin is essential as well.

Iron

Iron is an important element for blood health. It helps form hemoglobin, the part of red blood cells that brings oxygen to tissues and collects carbon dioxide waste and brings it to the lungs.

"Iron-deficiency" anemia describes the result of not having enough iron to ensure this pickup and delivery system is in good working order. Fatigue, weakness, pale skin, and headaches are the main signs of anemia, though iron deficiency is not the only possible cause. Anemia must be diagnosed by a doctor and the underlying cause identified and treated.

Adults over 50 years of age need 10 mg of iron daily, as do children up to age 10. But females from age 11 to 50 need 15 mg, and pregnant women need 30 mg. This is because between puberty and menopause, women menstruate monthly, and iron is needed to replenish the supply of blood lost. Menstruation does not occur during pregnancy, but the volume of the mother's blood is increased markedly to nourish the growing fetus.

Good sources of iron are beef (especially beef liver), fish, poultry, shellfish, eggs, legumes, dried fruits, and iron-fortified cereals.

Iodine

Iodine is used by the body to make thyroid hormones, which regulate metabolism. It also has an important role in fetal development. Iodine is available in needed amounts in seafood and, as the name suggests, in iodized salt.

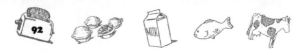

People who eat little saltwater fish or other seafood or use salt that has not been iodized are at risk for iodine deficiency.

The sign of this is a goiter, an enlargement of the thyroid that shows up as a large lump at the front of the neck. A child born of a mother with iodine deficiency may suffer from cretinism, a birth defect that is characterized by mental and physical retardation.

Adults and children over the age of 11 years need 150 mcg of iodine a day, an amount readily available from normal usage of iodized salt. Women need 175 mcg during pregnancy and 200 mcg during breastfeeding.

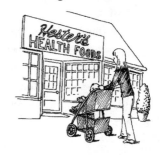

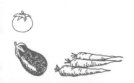

Fluoride

Fluoride plays an important role in bone and tooth formation. Throughout childhood, adequate amounts of fluoride are required for both. To respond to this need, many municipalities add safe levels of fluoride to the public water supply. Children who live in areas where water is not fluoridated often suffer from severe dental caries (cavities) and poorly formed bones unless they take supplementary fluoride, which requires a doctor's prescription.

Tea and seafood are other sources of fluoride, but fluoridated drinking water is by far the most reliable. Adults and teenagers need between 3 and 4 mg of fluoride daily. The amount needed for younger children varies with their age. If you are uncertain whether your

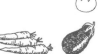

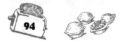

growing child is getting enough fluoride, talk to
your pediatrician.

The Special Case of Salt

Salt is a compound consisting of
sodium and chlorine, two of the major
essential minerals. Their role is to help
maintain the proper fluid balance in cells
of the body.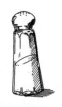

Adults need 500 mg of sodium each day
and 750 mg of chlorine. It is the rare person
who doesn't get more than that.

We get most of our sodium and chlorine
from table salt, which we add to food while
cooking or at the dining table. Soy sauce is
loaded with it. Many fresh foods contain some
salt, as does water, and prepared foods, especially snack and fast foods, contain a lot. Even

milk and yogurt contain salt, 120 mg and 160 mg per cup respectively, and cheese can contain as much as 400 mg of salt per ounce. Take a look at the label of foods you regularly buy and eat. You will be amazed at how much salt even apparently unsalty foods contain.

The fact is, most of us should be reducing our salt intake. The current recommendation is that people get no more than 2,400 mg of sodium daily. (One teaspoon of salt contains 2,000 mg of sodium.) People who have or are at risk for high blood pressure are urged to reduce their salt intake to far below that because of the association between high blood pressure and sodium.

"Association" does not mean a proven cause-and-effect relationship, but it does mean that high sodium intake has been observed in many people with high blood pressure and that reducing sodium intake can help lower it.

The connection between sodium and blood pressure is the subject of controversy, and until it has been solved, it's a good idea to limit salt intake by:

- Not adding salt to food on your plate
- Relying on other flavor enhancers such as herbs and spices when cooking
- Going easy on cured and pickled foods, since salt is used in the preserving process
- Limiting luncheon and deli meats, which are high in fat as well as salt
- Choosing low-salt or salt-free alternatives when you eat canned soups and vegetables, or use soy sauce
- Snacking on more unsalted and low-salt foods (fresh fruits and vegetables, for example) than on pretzels, chips, salty crackers, and salted popcorn

There really is no danger of developing a sodium or chlorine deficiency, given the typical American diet, so going easy on salt will do no harm and may even help. Talk with your doctor if you want to know more about how this applies to you.

Are Vitamin and Mineral Supplements Necessary?

When it comes to children, and especially babies, vitamin and mineral supplements are not necessary and may not even be safe.

Children need far lower amounts of micronutrients than adults and probably get as much as they need in the food they eat. Babies who are breastfed by mothers who are well nourished will

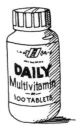

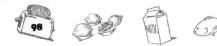

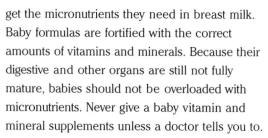

get the micronutrients they need in breast milk. Baby formulas are fortified with the correct amounts of vitamins and minerals. Because their digestive and other organs are still not fully mature, babies should not be overloaded with micronutrients. Never give a baby vitamin and mineral supplements unless a doctor tells you to.

Once your children start eating solid foods, their growing bodies and maturing organs will get what they need from the variety of foods you introduce. If you are worried that your children might not be getting enough, focus on smart nutrition: Make sure they are eating a balanced diet, which will provide them with the vitamins and minerals they need, as well as appropriate amounts of fat, protein, and carbohydrate.

Children's vitamins tend to be flavored and marketed as yummy treats, so there is a danger than an unattended child will eat them like candy. In fact, there is a much greater risk of a child getting too much, rather than too little. Vitamin and mineral tablets for children are a waste of money at best and could be worse than that.

To be absolutely safe, treat vitamin and mineral supplements like medicine:

- Keep them out of the reach and sight of children.
- Keep them in containers with childproof covers.
- Never refer to them as candy or offer them as a treat.
- If you suspect a child has eaten more than a single vitamin pill in a day, call your local poison control center without delay.

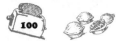

If you are really concerned about a deficiency—if your child is a picky eater and you can't seem to get his or her diet in balance, or if he or she suffers from a metabolic disorder that interferes with absorption of nutrients and micronutrients—talk with your child's doctor.

Adults need more micronutrients than children, but a balanced diet is still the best way to go. There are exceptions, however:

- Women of all ages need supplemental calcium to prevent osteoporosis. At least 400 IU (10 mcg) of vitamin D should be taken at the same time. There are several different forms of calcium. Calcium citrate is thought to be easier for the body to absorb and less likely to cause heartburn and constipation than calcium carbonate.

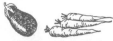

- Folate deficiency in early pregnancy can result in spina bifida and other neural tube defects in babies. These birth defects cripple and kill. Supplements taken after conception may be too late to prevent defects. That is why it is recommended that all females of childbearing age (from puberty to menopause) take supplements to ensure they get 400 mcg daily and 600 mcg while pregnant.

Most daily supplements contain enough folic acid, though not enough calcium. There is no harm in taking a single multivitamin/mineral each day. But I urge you to leave it at that.

Taking single element supplements or large doses is wasteful and can be risky. For water-soluble vitamins, taking more than your body can use is a bit like dumping them down the drain. With fat-soluble vitamins, which are not readily eliminated in the urine, there is the danger of building up toxic levels. The same goes for minerals, some of which can be toxic when taken in excess.

There are several health conditions that make it difficult to absorb or process certain micronutrients. These include kidney disease (and dialysis), metabolic and digestive disorders, HIV, and cancer. Chronic alcoholism, diet addiction, and other eating disorders often go hand in hand with nutritional deficiencies. Elderly people may be more prone to deficiencies as well, and women who are pregnant or breastfeeding their babies also have different nutritional needs. Some prescription medications interact with vitamins, interfering with the body's ability to use them.

If any of these conditions apply to you or if, for other reasons, you suspect you might have a vitamin or mineral deficiency, talk with your doctor, who can check if you have symptoms or signs of a particular deficiency and discuss with you ways to adjust your diet and/or use supplements to make up what is lacking.

For the rest of us, food is the best source of micronutrients. If you're smart about nutrition, chances are you'll get all the vitamins and minerals you need.

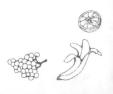

What Else Is Food Made Of?

There are two other components of food, both liquid. One you don't need at all, and one you need more than anything else that goes in your mouth.

Alcohol

The one you do not need is alcohol, a product of carbohydrate fermentation. It exists in minute amounts in many foods and in quite large amounts in some beverages—wine, beer, liquor, and the like. Each gram of alcohol supplies seven calories. Unlike fat, protein, and carbohydrates, however, it provides no nutritional benefit. As a food, alcohol is of no value, though it can certainly add to a weight problem. For some people it is worse than that. Alcohol has both short- and long-term effects on the brain and nervous system, altering response time, mood, and body chemistry. It can be addictive, with far-reaching negative effects.

Some studies suggest that moderate amounts of some alcoholic beverages, especially red wine, might confer some health benefits. This is largely because of chemicals other than alcohol contained in them. The jury is still out on this, however, so consuming alcohol cannot be recommended as a smart nutrition choice.

Water

It's colorless, odorless, flavorless. It has no fat,
protein, or carbohydrates, and no calories
either. Still, it's the most important element in
your diet and you probably aren't getting
enough of it.

You can go a month or more without food,
and live to tell the tale. But a few days without
water will kill you. That's a simple fact.

Most foods contain at least some water,
and some foods contain a lot of it. Fruits and
vegetables get their juiciness from water, and
juices obviously do. Milk is
mostly water. Coffee, tea,
and soft drinks are essen-
tially flavored water, though
they contain lots of chemicals and often contain sugar
as well. And some of those

chemicals actually draw water out of cells rather than putting it in. But even with all this water, everyone needs lots of just plain water, with nothing added.

Smart nutrition includes drinking a minimum of eight 8-ounce glasses of water each day. That's 64 ounces, two quarts, a half gallon. More won't hurt you. But it should be water. Not coffee or tea or juice or soda or beer. Water, plain and simple.

Why Do You Need Water?

Water makes up at least 50 percent of your body, and fully 80 percent of your blood, 70 percent of your muscles, and a whopping 85 percent of your brain! In addition, water plays a major role in a wide range of body processes. It:

- Helps regulate your body temperature

- Carries nutrients to your cells
- Keeps your skin supple, your eyes, nose, mouth, and internal organs moist
- Provides cushioning for your joints
- Is the major component of tears and saliva
- Removes wastes from your body through urine and sweat
- Helps keep your bowels moving, especially if you are eating more fiber (which you should be) since soluble fiber can be constipating.
- Dissolves vitamins, minerals, and other nutrients so your body can use them

I could go on, but you get the general idea.

The average person loses about 10 cups (that's 80 ounces) of water a day through sweat, exhaling, and urine and feces. That water has to be replaced. That's why you can't rely merely on water in food and beverages.

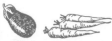

You need to chug at least 64 ounces of plain old H_2O.

How Can You Be Sure You Get Enough Water?

It's hard to get in the habit of drinking enough water, but here are some tips to help you do it:

- Fill a half gallon bottle or pitcher with water and put it in your refrigerator every morning. If it's empty by the time you go to bed, you've had your daily dose. (This works only if no one else is drinking out of that bottle, but you get the idea.)
- Fill several small plastic water bottles a quarter of the way and put them in the freezer. Every time you or a member of your family goes out—to work, to school, to play—

top off the bottle, slip it into a gym sock (to keep it from sweating and make it more pleasant to hold), and send it along. Sip until it's empty and then refill it at any fountain or faucet.

- When eating out, order water first thing, and drink it while you read the menu and wait for your meal.

- Every time you're thirsty, think (and drink) water first and other beverages second.

- Get into the habit of drinking a glass of water before each meal, upon waking, and before you go to sleep.

- In hot weather or if you are exercising heavily, drink water *before* you feel thirsty. You are losing water through sweat, but by the time you are thirsty, you are nearing dehydration.

The very young and the very old are at greater risk of dehydration than the rest of us.

- Be sure your babies and toddlers drink plenty of water. You may have more wet diapers, but they'll also be starting a good habit early in life.
- If you are elderly or are caring for someone who is, schedule a water break at least every hour or two.

Now you know what food is made of. The next step to smart nutrition is to learn how you can make the most of it.

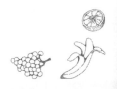

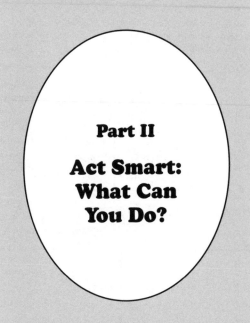

Part II

Act Smart: What Can You Do?

The Food Guide Pyramid

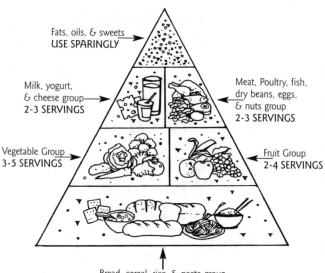

Fats, oils, & sweets
USE SPARINGLY

Milk, yogurt,
& cheese group
2-3 SERVINGS

Meat, Poultry, fish,
dry beans, eggs,
& nuts group
2-3 SERVINGS

Vegetable Group
3-5 SERVINGS

Fruit Group
2-4 SERVINGS

Bread, cereal, rice, & pasta group
6-11 SERVINGS

Find the Balance

J ust about everyone agrees that a balanced diet leads to smart nutrition, but how can you be sure that your diet is balanced? The USDA, which advises Americans on healthful eating, developed a way to illustrate a balanced diet: The Food Guide Pyramid.

The Food Guide Pyramid

The Food Guide Pyramid is based on research on what Americans eat, what nutrients are in

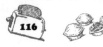

those foods, and how to make food choices that promote good health. One of the best things about the Food Guide Pyramid is that it works for every taste. By indicating types of foods rather than specific ones, it allows you to make choices according to what you like. Ethnic foods, prepared foods, health foods, diet foods, restaurant foods, snack foods—anything edible, in fact—has a place. You get to choose what makes your mouth water.

Even though the Food Guide Pyramid is not about calories, it can be used by people who want to lose weight. It's just a matter of choosing low-calorie foods from each part of the Pyramid. It does urge going easy on fats and sugars, which is good for dieters as well as the rest of us. But it is possible for anyone to get enough calories every day, and to avoid getting too many. It also works for people of any age.

As the pyramid, or triangular, shape suggests, foods at the bottom, the widest part, are those you should eat the most of. Those at the tip should be eaten as little as possible. Let's take a look at the specifics, starting from the top:

Sugar and Fats

This is the tip, or narrowest part of the pyramid, and the guidelines say, "Eat sparingly."

As you already know, it is recommended that no more than 30 percent of your total daily calorie intake come from fat, and of that not more than 10 percent should be saturated fat. Does that mean you can get up to 30 percent of your calories from butter, margarine, and oil you add to your food? No, absolutely not!

If you take a close look at the pyramid you'll see little specks and flakes all over the

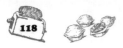

place. These are fats and sugars, and it's obvious that they can be found in foods in all categories. There is fat in meat and dairy products, for example, and to a lesser degree in some vegetables. Fruits are major sources of sugar. Bread, baked goods, and especially snack foods are sources of both fat and sugar.

Because most of us eat too much fat, it is important to be aware of the fat content of all the foods you eat. If your total is under 30 percent, you can think about adding a pat of butter or a squirt of oil, but "eat sparingly" is an excellent guideline. Likewise, remember that simple sugars are mostly "empty calories," and not the best way to get the carbohydrates you need.

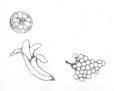

Meat, Fish, Poultry, Dairy, Eggs, Nuts, and Dried Beans (Legumes)

These are the major sources of protein in any diet. Vegetarians of any type as well as meat eaters will find good sources of protein on this second level. Remember, if 10 percent of your daily calories come from protein, you'll be getting as much as you need.

Note that dried beans and other legumes (lentils, split peas), as well as tofu, which is made from soybeans, can also be in the vegetable category, so if you've used your daily allotment from this group, you can count them as a vegetable serving.

Except for dried beans and tofu, all the foods on this level contain significant amounts of fat, so make your choices with that in mind. The guidelines say, "Eat two to three servings a day."

Fruit

The pyramid gets wider when it gets to fruits, which are a good source of vitamins and fiber. They are thirst-quenching and a dandy dessert alternative to cakes, cookies, and other sweets. Still, they *are* sweet, and that's because of the sugar they contain. Even though fruits are carbohydrate foods, they contain a lot of fructose, a simple sugar, which is not as good a choice as complex carbohydrates.

The guidelines recommend eating two to four servings a day.

Vegetables

Whether it's root vegetables like carrots and potatoes or leafy vegetables like lettuce

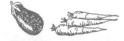

and spinach, any of the variety of squashes or members of the onion family (garlic, scallions, shallots, and more), or one of the many other edible plants, vegetables are an excellent source of vitamins. Most are also high in fiber, and all are low in fat.

These carbohydrate foods are such an important part of a balanced diet that they are just one step up from the widest part of the pyramid. The guidelines say, "Eat three to five servings a day."

Grains and Cereals

At the very bottom of the pyramid you'll find grain and grain products. This includes flours of every type and bread and the other baked goods made from them; pasta and noodles; rice of every variety; and breakfast cereals. These starchy foods and ingredients are the principal source of complex carbohydrates, the backbone of a healthful diet. Whole grains are also high in fiber, which is why they are recommended over refined flours and the foods made from them.

Fat, oils, and sugars are often combined with these, especially in breads, cakes, crackers, and many breakfast cereals, so you should be aware of the ingredients of the foods you choose. (Watch those little flecks scattered throughout the pyramid!)

Nonetheless, following the guidelines means eating some grain or cereal product at every meal in order to "Eat six to 11 servings a day."

What Is a Serving?

Using the Food Guide Pyramid requires understanding what a serving is. Strictly speaking, a serving is what the USDA has decided an average person eats. Who that average person is remains a mystery. You might eat more or less. What's important is that recommendations and calorie counts on food labels are all based on this theoretical average eater.

Here's how it translates:

Meat, Fish, Poultry, Eggs, Nuts, and Dried Beans

One serving equals:

- 2–3 ounces of cooked lean meat, poultry, or fish (Hint: That's about the size of a deck of cards.)
- 1 cup of cooked dry beans
- 2 eggs
- 7 ounces of tofu (soybean cake)
- 4 tablespoons of peanut or other nut butter
- ½ cup of nuts or seeds

Dairy (Milk, Yogurt, Cheese)

One serving equals:

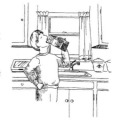

- 1 cup (8 ounces) of milk
- 1 cup (8 ounces) of yogurt
- 1½ ounces natural cheese
- 2 ounces processed cheese or "cheese food"
- 2 cups cottage cheese
- 1 cup ice cream or frozen yogurt

Fruits

One serving equals:

- 1 medium apple, orange, or banana
- ½ cup chopped, cooked, or canned fruit
- ¼ cup dried fruit
- ¾ cup (6 ounces) fruit juice

Vegetables

One serving equals:

- 1 cup raw leafy vegetables (lettuce, spinach, greens)
- ½ cup cooked or chopped raw of other vegetables
- ¾ cup (6 ounces) vegetable juice

Grains, Bread, Cereals, Rice, Pasta

One serving equals:

- 1 slice of bread
- 1 medium muffin, doughnut, or danish (about 2 ounces)
- ½ bagel, English muffin, or hamburger roll
- 3–4 crackers
- 1 ounce ready-to-eat cereal
- ½ cup cooked cereal
- ½ cup cooked rice
- ½ cup cooked pasta

You'll learn more about serving sizes and how to be smart about them at the supermarket, in the kitchen, and at the dining table in the next two chapters.

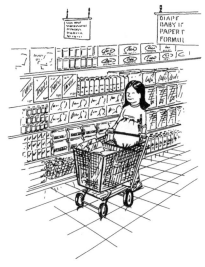

8 Shop Smart

The grocery store is the front line for anyone who wants to be smart about nutrition. What you buy, and don't buy, can make all the difference in what you and your family eat. If you shop according to the Food Guide Pyramid, chances are good you'll be eating that way too.

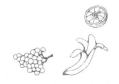

Make a List

Never go food shopping without a list. Whether you plan all meals in advance or like to have a variety of ingredients on hand so you can make meals to suit your mood, it's a good idea to write down what you need. Otherwise, you will be at the mercy of the food packagers, who arrange supermarket shelves to "push" the items they want to sell. Too often, these are sugar- and fat-laden foods.

Whether you shop in a supermarket, farmer's market, corner grocery store, or organic/health food store, fill your basket with whole grain breads, fresh fruits and vegetables, and low-fat dairy items. Go easy on fatty meats, especially luncheon meats, and sweet desserts.

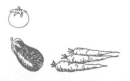

Be especially aware when you buy anything that is precooked, frozen, canned, or in a packaged mix. This is where the trans fats, saturated fats, and sugars hide. The lucky part about that is that these are also foods that are labeled.

Required Reading

According to the law, all packaged and prepared foods must carry nutritional information, including calorie content, on their labels. This includes foods that come in boxes, cans, bottles, and numerous other containers. Fresh fruits and vegetables, unprocessed meats, and other "unpackaged" foods are not included. Nonetheless, most of the foods Americans buy and eat are covered by the label law. Reading labels can give you a

lot of useful information, if you know how to
look for it.

Nutrition Facts	Amount/Serving	%DV*	Amount/Serving	%DV*
Serv. Size ½ cup (120 mL) condensed soup	**Total Fat** 2g	3%	**Potassium** 260mg	7%
	Sat. Fat 0.5g	3%	**Total Carb.** 9g	3%
Servings about 2 ½	Polyunsat. Fat 0.5g		Fiber 0g	
Calories 70	Monounsat. Fat 1g		Sugars 1g	
Fat Cal. 20	**Cholest.** 15mg	5%	**Protein** 3g	
*Percent Daily Values (DV) are based on a 2,000 calorie diet.	**Sodium** 480mg	20%		
	Vitamin A 10 % • Vitamin C 0% • Calcium 0% • Iron 4%			

- Serving size is perhaps the most important
  piece of information you will find on a
  label. Except for single-serving items, food
  packages contain more than one serving.
  The first two lines on the approved food
  label tell you the size of a serving and the
  number of servings in the package.
- Calorie content is the next important piece
  of data. The number of calories indicated is

always *per serving,* not per package. You can determine the number of calories in the whole package by multiplying calories by number of servings. That's a good way to find out how many calories you are actually eating (or drinking) if you "eat the whole thing!"

- The label also tells you the number of grams, *per serving,* of fat, protein, and carbohydrate.

- Fat is given as total fat and saturated fat, *per serving,* but monounsaturated, polyunsaturated, and trans fats are not singled out according to regulations now in effect.

- Carbohydrates are given as total grams, *per serving.* Fiber and sugar are broken out. To find out how many grams of complex carbohydrate there are in each serving, subtract the fiber and sugar from the total.

- Because consumption of cholesterol and salt (sodium) are health concerns for many people, the grams *per serving* of these are listed as well.

- The label also tells the percentage of daily value of each component. These percentages are based on a 2,000-calorie diet, so your own daily allotment may differ.

- Vitamins and minerals that exist in significant amounts are listed as well, along with the percentage of them in the "typical" 2,000-calorie diet.

Sniffing Out the Bad Guys

Ingredients are listed on the food label in order of their weight. That is, the earlier in the list an ingredient appears, the more (by weight) there is of it. This is where manufacturers may try to pull the wool over your eyes. But if you know their tricks, you won't be fooled.

The two areas where the label writers can fudge are sugar and fats, especially when it comes to those stealthy trans fats.

If you look for any words that say "fat" to you, and you find them close to the bottom of the list, you might think there isn't much fat in that particular food. In fact, fat goes by many names, and most packaged foods contain more than one type. A single food might contain butter, lard, hydrogenated and partially hydrogenated vegetable oils (that's where your trans fats are), fish oils, shortening, and any number of fat-containing ingredients, such as lecithin, milk, eggs, and more. Small amounts (by weight)

of many different fats can be used to hide the true story of the fat content. The way to unmask these ingredients is to look back at the fat content part of the label.

As for sugar, look for these sugar aliases:

- brown sugar
- corn sweetener
- corn syrup
- fructose
- fruit juice concentrate
- glucose
- dextrose
- high-fructose corn syrup

- honey
- invert sugar
- lactose
- maltose
- molasses
- raw sugar
- sucrose
- syrup

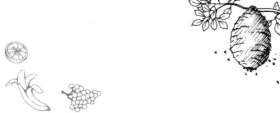

If the label is bottom-loaded with several of these, you can be sure there's a lot of sugar in the food. Check the sugar content by gram and the truth will emerge.

Decoding Labeling Terms

People who are smart about nutrition may look for the terms low fat, reduced fat, no fat, low calorie, reduced calorie, and light (or lite) when they are making food selections. But what do these terms mean? The short answer is that they do not necessarily mean a food is low in fat or a smart nutrition choice in other ways. The long answer comes from the FDA, which has set strict rules about the use of these terms:

- **Free** means that a product contains no amount of, or only trivial amounts of, fat,

saturated fat, cholesterol, sodium, sugars,
and/or calories.

- **Low (or Lo)** means the food can be eaten
  frequently without exceeding dietary guidelines for fat, saturated fat, cholesterol,
  sodium, and/or calories. According to this
  definition, low calorie means 40 calories or
  fewer per serving; low fat means 3 grams
  or fewer per serving.

- **Reduced** means that the product contains at
  least 25 percent less of a nutrient or of
  calories than the regular product. However,
  a reduced claim can't be made on a
  product if the regular version meets the
  requirement for a "low" claim. For example,
  all pretzels are low in fat, so a particular
  brand of pretzels cannot be termed
  "reduced fat." And calling them low fat

does not make them low calorie! Pretzels get their calories from carbohydrates, at the rate of four calories per gram.

- **Less** means that a food contains 25 percent less of a nutrient or of calories than the regular version. For example, pretzels that have 25 percent less fat than potato chips could carry a "less" claim.

- **Light (or Lite)** means that a product contains one third fewer calories or half the fat of the regular version. If the food derives 50 percent or more of its calories from fat, the reduction must be 50 percent of the fat.

Be aware, though, that "light" can also be used to refer to salt (sodium) content and to describe such properties as texture and color, as long as the label explains the intent—for

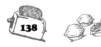

example, "light brown sugar" and "light and fluffy."

Now that you know how to shop smart, the next step is to take the food home and prepare it in a way to spells smart nutrition for everyone who eats it.

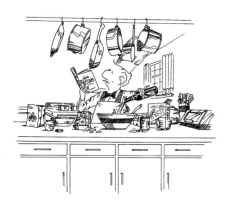

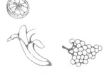

9 Eat Smart

The cornerstone of smart eating is cutting down on fat. If you do nothing else, you'll be doing a lot, for your health and that of your family. Almost without trying, you will end up eating more carbohydrates, and will get enough protein with little effort. The same goes for the vitamins and minerals you need.

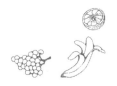

140

Cut the Fat

Whether you are overweight, underweight, or just
the weight you should be, whether or not you
have health problems associated with high-fat
eating; whether you cook for yourself or for a
family that includes growing children who are
now in tip-top shape, you should focus on eating
less fat. Your goals should be:

- No more than 30 percent of daily calories
  from fat. If you want to know how this
  applies to you and your family, look at the
  "Recommended Fat Intake" chart in
  Chapter 10
- Less than that if you want to lose weight,
  if you have high cholesterol, or any other
  health problem associated with a
  high-fat diet

- Less than one-third of your daily fat should be saturated, the kind of fat found in animal products (meat and dairy)
- The remaining two-thirds (20 percent of your daily calorie intake) should be from unsaturated fats, with an emphasis on monounsaturated fats (olive, canola, and peanut oils)

You can accomplish this through a combination of strategies, whether you cook and eat at home most of the time or often eat out. If you are the meal planner and cook in your household, you can have a major influence on the eating habits and health of the people you live with, young and old.

How Many Meals Should You Eat?

The classic "three square meals a day" may be more myth than reality. Aside from breakfast, lunch, and dinner, snacks make up a significant part of what most people eat during the day. And let's be honest: A snack is a meal. Even those who skip breakfast (not a good idea) tend to nibble their way to lunchtime.

Snacking in and of itself is not a bad thing. Having many small meals is no less healthful than having three larger ones. The secret is to be aware of what you're eating and make smart choices.

No matter how many meals you eat, the total number of calories you take in should be what you need to maintain a healthy weight. The components of those meals should represent the

balance we have talked about. Be guided by the
Food Guide Pyramid and the warnings about fat.
And every meal, or snack, or break in the day
should be looked upon as an opportunity to
have a glass of water.

Home on the Range (and in the Fridge)

Cooking and eating at home gives you the
most control over what you and others in
your household eat. It begins with making
sure the refrigerator and cup-
boards are filled with smart
nutrition choices.
Remember, if you
don't buy it, you
won't eat it.

Here are some things you can do:

- Fill your refrigerator with fresh fruits and vegetables, and a bottomless jug of drinking water.
- Arrange food in the refrigerator so the smart choices are front and center, and the dangerous temptations are buried in the back.
- Once a week, take everything out of the refrigerator/freezer and take a hard look at the high-fat foods that crept in there over the previous week. See if you can discard some of them and work on making sure you (and others who have the "key" to the fridge) don't let them in again. The password to your refrigerator and freezer should be: "Phooey on fat!"

- Stock your cupboard with whole-grain breads and crisps. Choose flat breads and other crunchy snacks rather than chips and trans fat-heavy crackers.
- Sprinkle sesame and sunflower seeds on salads and vegetables
- Sweeten breakfast cereals with fruit instead of sugar.
- When planning desserts, think about a bowl of cut-up fresh fruit with a dollop of yogurt rather than a bowl of ice cream with a dollop of fruit syrup.
- Use a frother to whip up low-fat milk for your coffee instead of using cream.
- Snack smart on carrot and celery sticks, rings of sweet pepper, and rounds of cucumber

dipped in spicy salsa, instead of salty chips and a creamy dip.

- Tempt your kids with an after-school snack of apple slices spread with peanut butter instead of milk and cookies.

In short, concentrate on complex carbohydrates, including fiber, and turn away from fat, sugar, and salt.

Substitute

Trade in high-fat choices and go for low-fat ones. For example:

- Use skim and 1 percent milk instead of 2 percent and whole milk.
- Use yogurt instead of sour cream on baked potatoes and in dips.

- Use low- or no-fat cottage and other cheeses.
- Shun mayonnaise in favor of ketchup and mustard
- Squeeze lemon juice over vegetables instead of butter or margarine
- Overstuff sandwiches with lettuce, sprouts, and other crunchy vegetables, and go easy on the meat
- Use tuna and other canned fish packed in water instead of oil

Now You're Cookin'

The way you cook food is nearly as important as what you cook when it comes to reducing fat and pre-serving nutrients.

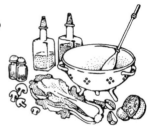

Begin by trimming the fat off all meat you plan to cook. Here are some easy ways to do it:

- Use scissors or a sharp knife to trim fat surrounding steak, chops, and other cuts of meat before you cook them.
- It's often easier to remove fat from meat when it is frozen.
- Remove skin from chicken and fish before cooking.
- Refrigerate gravy and broth and then lift off the layer of fat that forms on the top.

Choose cooking methods that require little or no added fat and remove existing fat in the process. Here are some easy ways to do it:

- Grill, broil, or roast meat on a rack, with a pan beneath it to catch the fat.

- When making gravy, pour off all fat from the drippings. Use a special fat separator, a bulb baster, or float a paper towel over the surface to absorb the fat.

- Steam or microwave foods to keep them moist and to preserve water-soluble vitamins.

- Try nonstick spray rather than butter or other shortening to keep food from sticking to the pan.

- Use nonstick pans and a small amount of unsaturated oil to sauté or stir-fry foods.

- Save stews, heavy gravies, and cream sauces for the occasional meal, and forget about deep frying. In time, you and the people you cook for will lose the

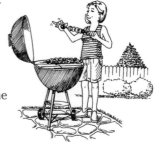

taste for these very rich preparations, and
may not miss them at all.

Pay Attention to Serving Size

It's all well and good to read food labels and
cook the low-fat way, but if you do not also pay
attention to how many servings you and your
family are eating, you're still not eating smart.

Most packaged food contains more than one
serving and so do most home recipes. The food
label will tell you not only what is considered a
single serving of that food ("serving size"), but
also how many servings the package contains.
Most recipes tell you how many people it serves.

But how many of you munch mindlessly
from an open box of crackers or chips and still
tell yourself you've eaten only one serving? How

many cut an extra-large slice of cake or pie and call it a single portion, or forget to add "seconds" when thinking about your daily intake of calories and fat? How many of you cooks sample what you're making and down that last morsel while cleaning up after a meal? Don't all raise your hands at the same time, but do think about breaking the freelance tasting habit and measuring servings until portion control becomes second nature to you.

You can measure servings in various ways. Sometimes it is a matter of counting pieces. Other times a measuring cup, spoon, or kitchen scale will give you the information you need. For packaged food, it may be a matter of dividing the contents into the number of servings it contains, and eating only one portion. After a while, you will have a pretty good idea of what a

serving of a particular food looks like. Still, it is a
good idea to start out by measuring and go back
to measuring every once in a while.

Away from Home

It's a whole lot easier to eat smart at home than it
is when you're away. The same goes for the rest
of your family. But everyone in your household can
be a smart brown-bagger by adopting these habits:

- Eat breakfast, and eat it at home. It's far too
  easy to skip this vital meal, which you need
  after the longest between-meals break of your
  entire day. Make it a balanced meal, with
  enough of each of the nutrient groups to hold
  you until lunchtime. A donut and coffee is not
  a balanced breakfast, and a fast-food breakfast
  sandwich is another way to spell F-A-T.

- Whenever possible, pack your lunch. Luncheonettes, salad bars, and fast food restaurants are expensive in more ways than one. High-fat and salty foods are staples there.

- Bagged lunch doesn't have to mean nothing but sandwiches. All you need to pack soups and salads are plastic containers with close-fitting lids, and a refrigerator and/or microwave at your workplace.

- Pack a snack of nuts, seeds, and dried fruit, or fresh fruit, along with lunch. That way, donuts and candy bars won't be tempting when energy starts to lag in the midmorning or mid-afternoon.

- Bring along a water bottle, and fill it often throughout the day.

Restaurant Rescue

Eating in restaurants can be a minefield, but here's a map to help you get through it:

- Make eating out a special occasion, not an everyday habit.
- Avoid fast food restaurants, and any place that boasts an all-you-can eat menu, buffets, or oversized meals
- Choose restaurants that feature low-fat cuisines. Instead of the local steakhouse or pizza parlor, try eateries that specialize in Chinese and Asian foods and fish and other seafood.

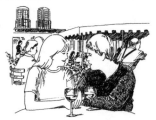

Wherever you go, order wisely:

- Drink a glass of water while you read the menu, and push the butter and bread basket to the other side of the table, or ask that they be taken away.
- Begin with a salad, soup, or fruit course, which will quell your appetite before you get to the main event.
- Choose dishes that are baked, boiled, grilled, poached, steamed, or raw, rather than stews and fried foods. That includes boiled or baked potatoes instead of mashed or french fried.
- Ask that sauces, gravies, and dressings be served on the side, and then add only a bit.
- Ask for vegetables served without butter.
- Say "yes" to the pepper grinder but "no, thanks" to the grated cheese.

- When it comes to dessert, consider skipping it, or order fresh fruit or sorbet. If you really can't resist, share a dessert with your dining companions. A small piece or a spoonful will give you a taste without breaking your fat bank, and it may satisfy your curiosity and craving for the double chocolate mousse cake with ganache icing.

Party Time

Parties and holiday gatherings are a challenge to smart nutrition. Here are some damage control hints:

- Front load your smart nutrition choices. On party days, make every other meal a low-fat one. Concentrate on vegetables and complex carbohydrates, and drink a lot of water. Chances are, you'll be spending your fat and

sugar allowance at the party, so under eat
from the upper part of the Food Guide
Pyramid before you get to the party.

- As soon as you arrive, get something to
  drink. A sugar-free soda or seltzer with a slice
  of lime is a good choice. If you want something stronger, think about a wine spritzer.
  Nurse your drink. And be aware that among
  its other undesirable features, alcohol reduces
  your inhibitions and may make it harder for
  you to be smart about what you eat.

- When the hors d'oeuvres tray makes its
  appearance, make yourself scarce. If you really
  can't resist, go for the raw veggies. Whatever
  you do, do not pick up a plate and fill it with
  nibbles—take everything piece by piece.

- If the meal is a buffet, take a small plate and
  fill it with vegetables and other carbohydrates,

go easy on the protein, and forget the sauce. If you get at the end of the line, you'll be one of the last to sit down and less likely to go back for seconds.

- If it's a sit-down meal, say "no, thank you" to sauce and gravy, ask for a modest portion, and forget about seconds.

- Be the first one up to help clear the table. You'll not only make points with your host, but you'll be away from the table and out of the minefield.

- At every social or family gathering, concentrate on the people there rather than the food. Good conversation does a great job of distracting you from the fried wontons and sour cream dip!

Smart Dieting

This is not a book about weight loss. But because dieting is a subject of intense and continuing interest to many Americans, I do want to say a few words.

- The only way to lose weight is to take in fewer calories than your body needs.
- The safe way to do that is gradually, changing your eating habits over the course of time. Quick weight loss inevitably is followed by quick weight gain.
- The smart way to do it is with a combination of eating less (taking in fewer calories) and exercising more (using more calories).
- When you cut fat, you automatically reduce

your intake of a nutrient that supplies more than twice the number of calories as carbohydrate and protein.

- Use the Food Guide Pyramid to give shape to your weight-loss plans. Eating a balanced diet is important, especially when you are taking in fewer calories.

- Get support for your weight-loss plan. Family and friends, support groups, and tools like food and activity journals, calorie counters, and fat gram counters can make all the difference. *The Everything® Calorie Mini Book* and *The Everything® Fat Gram Mini Book* are two good sources of nutritional information.

A Word About Eating Disorders

Before you decide to lose weight, make sure you really need to. Check your body mass index

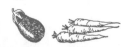

(see Chapter 10). If it is over 25, you should lose weight, but if it is below 18, you definitely should not, no matter how fat you think you are. For would-be dieters with BMIs near and below 18, discuss your feelings about being overweight with your doctor and take a look at the website of the American Anorexia Bulimia Association (*www.aabainc.org*).

Food Safety

America has the world's safest food supply, yet every once in a while we hear news about food poisoning and contamination. Whether you eat at home or at a restaurant or other public eatery, the possibility of becoming ill from food is a concern.

Food can be contaminated with bacteria, fungi, and parasites. In some cases, the living organisms are benign. For example, yogurt and cheese owe their existence to bacteria, and blue-veined cheeses and mushrooms are all about mold and fungi. In other cases, a healthy immune system can fight food contamination. Nonetheless, people do get sick, and sometimes die, when what they eat is spoiled or worse.

Two different bacteria, e. coli and salmonella, seem to get most of the attention.

- **E. coli** is a kind of bacteria that exists in all of our bodies. One particular strain of it, called 0157:H7, can make people really sick, however. It gets into food that has been touched by someone who did not wash his or her hands thoroughly. The contamination could have occurred as far away as the farm or processing plant or as close as a restaurant kitchen or even your own.

Heat kills bacteria, so the best way to protect against E. coli is to make sure the food you eat is fully cooked. E. coli has also been found in unpasteurized apple juice and lettuce, however, so cooking until well-done won't do in those cases. It is a good idea to avoid unpasteurized juice, and to give lettuce, as well as all other vegetables to be eaten raw, a good washing.

- **Salmonella** can be found in raw or undercooked eggs, poultry, meat, seafood, and dairy products. As with E. coli, heat will kill it, so the safest thing is to eat only thoroughly cooked food and pasteurized dairy products. Be particularly careful about eggs, which are the most frequent source of salmonella contamination. Do not eat raw eggs, but also do not taste cake and cookie batters, or let your children "lick the bowl or spoon," as happy a childhood memory as that may be for you.

Fight BAC

That's the motto of the government food safety program aimed at eliminating bacteria as a major source of food poisoning. Here are some smart kitchen habits that will help make your kitchen a safe place:

- While shopping, separate raw meat, poultry, and seafood from other food in your shopping cart. At check-out, have them placed in individual plastic bags and then bagged separately from other foods.
- When you unpack at home, put all meat, poultry, fish, and dairy products in the

refrigerator first. Make sure all are in containers or plastic bags so they don't drip on other foods.

- Store eggs in their original cartons (not in the egg tray of the refrigerator) and refrigerate them as soon as possible.

- Wash your hands with soap and warm water before and after you handle food, and often while preparing it. As a rule of thumb, wash your hands whenever you have handled raw meat and are about to handle another kind of food, especially one that will be eaten raw or lightly cooked.

- When cooking or otherwise handling food, be sure to wash your hands with soap and warm water after you use the bathroom, change a diaper, or touch your pets.

- Use paper towels to wipe up spills and dry your hands, then discard them after use. If you use cloth towels, wash them in the hot cycle of your washing machine; if you use sponges, put them in the dishwasher at the end of each day, and replace them often.

- Always use a clean cutting board. Wash the board and any knives with hot soapy water after preparing each food item, before you go on to the next.

- To be extra safe, use a different cutting board for meat, poultry, and fish than the one you use for vegetables and fruits. Color coding your cutting boards will help: red for meat and green for produce.

- Cook all meat, poultry, and shellfish thoroughly; use a thermometer to check internal temperature of roasts and whole poultry.
- Keep your refrigerator at 41 degrees Fahrenheit or cooler, and your freezer at zero degrees Fahrenheit.
- Always marinate food in the refrigerator; never use the marinade on cooked food unless you have boiled it just before serving.
- Refrigerate or freeze leftovers within two hours of cooking.
- Reheat leftovers until they are steaming hot.
- Pay attention to "sell by" dates, especially on all meat and dairy products you buy.
- Most leftovers should not be kept more than three or four days in the refrigerator or more than six months in the freezer.

- If you are in doubt about whether any food is spoiled or has been contaminated, throw it away.
- When packing food to go on a picnic, in a lunch box, or to the office, avoid mayonnaise, which contains raw eggs.
- If possible, pack food in a cooler. If not, include a frozen gel pack, juice box, or water bottle to keep food cool.
- When brown-bagging it in very hot weather, choose nonperishable foods such as peanut butter-and-jelly rather than meat or tuna or egg salad.

Given how much food we eat in a lifetime, the chances of any one person getting food poisoning are slight. Still, these precautions are worth taking. Food poisoning can be very serious for children, the elderly, pregnant women, and anyone with a weakened immune system. Anyone who develops fever, abdominal pain, vomiting, nausea, and diarrhea (especially if it is bloody) that cannot otherwise be explained should see a doctor.

Nutrition is a big subject and this is a small book. I've tried to tell you the most important things you need to know to be smart about nutrition, but I couldn't tell you everything. The next chapter will help you fill in the blanks by pointing you to other sources of information about this endlessly fascinating, and important, subject.

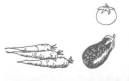

10 Get Smarter

There's a lot of information about nutrition available in books, magazines, and newsletters, on the Internet, and from health-focused associations and the federal government. Here is a list of some interesting sources, many of which will provide you with links and leads to others. At the end of this chapter, you will find some other smart nutrition tools, and a glossary of terms used in this book.

Smart Nutrition Resources
Associations and Government Agencies

American Anorexia Bulimia Association
165 West 46 Street, Suite 1108
New York, NY 10036
212-575-6200
www.aabainc.org
   Information and support on eating disorders

American Diabetes Association
1701 North Beauregard Street
Alexandria, VA 22311
800-DIABETES
www.diabetes.org
   Information about diabetes, but also excellent
   tips on healthful eating for all

American Dietetic Association
216 West Jackson Boulevard
Chicago, IL 60606
800-366-1655
www.eatright.org
   Recipes, information, and links

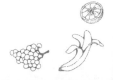

American Heart Association
7272 Greenville Avenue
Dallas, TX 75231
800-AHA-USA1
www.americanheart.org
Tips on heart healthy nutrition, among other
health strategies

 U.S. Department of Agriculture (USDA)
Food and Nutrition Information Center
National Agricultural Library, Room 304
10301 Baltimore Avenue
Beltsville, MD 20705
301-504-5719
www.nal.usda.gov/fnic
A treasure trove of information, databases,
publications, and links

 Consumer Information Center
Department WW, P.O. Box 100
Pueblo, CO 81009
800-688-9889
www.pueblo.gsa.gov/food.htm
Pamphlets and information sheets to order
or download on a wide range of food and
nutrition topics

Food and Drug Administration (FDA)
Center for Food Safety and Applied Nutrition
200 C Street SW
Washington, DC 20204
http://vm.cfsan.fda.gov
   Another treasure trove, your tax dollars
   at work for you

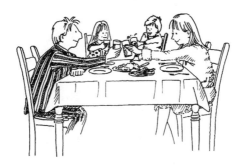

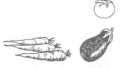

Booklets, Pamphlets, and Information Sheets

This is a small selection of informational material that can be ordered, for no or low cost, by mail or online. Some can even be downloaded from the organization's Web site (see the previous list for addresses).

✉ **From the American Dietetic Association**
Food Strategies for Men
Good Nutrition Reading List
The New Cholesterol Countdown
Staying Healthy—A Guide for Elder Americans

✉ **From the American Heart Association**
Easy Food Tips for Heart Healthy Eating
The AHA Diet: An Eating Plan for Healthy Americans
Nutritious Nibbles: A Guide to Healthy Snacking

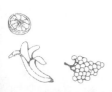

✉ From the Consumer Information Center

Action Guide for Healthy Eating
Bulking Up Fiber's Healthful Reputation
Dietary Guidelines for Americans 2000
Eat Right to Help Lower Your High Blood
  Pressure
Eating for Life
Fruits & Vegetables: Eating Your Way to 5 a Day
Growing Older, Eating Better
Snack Smart for Healthy Teeth

✉ From Iowa State University, Cooperative Extension Services

Cancer and Your Diet
Cholesterol in Your Body
Family Nutrition Guide
How to Eat Out Without Raising
  Your Cholesterol
Questions and Answers About Fat in
Your Diet
Questions and Answers About Sodium
  in Your Diet
Time Out for Facts About Foods,
  Fluids, and Athletic Performance for
  Teen Athletes Vegetarian Diets

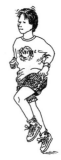

176

Newsletters

 Mayo Clinic Health Letter
PO Box 53889
Boulder, CO 80322
800-333-9037
www.healthestore.com/MayoNews/My_News_Hlx.asp

 Nutrition Action Health Letter
Center for Science in the Public Interest
1875 Connecticut Avenue, NW, Suite 300
Washington, DC 20009
www.cspinet.org

 Tufts University Health & Nutrition Letter
PO Box 57843
Boulder, CO 80321
800-274-7581
www.healthletter.tufts.edu

 **University of California, Berkeley
Wellness Letter**
Health Letter Associates
PO Box 420-235
Palm Coast, FL 32142
800-829-9080
www.berkeleywellness.com

Web Sites

In addition to the Web addresses given in the previous listings, surfing the following will yield lots of reliable information and valuable links to other Web sites.

Blonz Guide to Nutrition
A huge collection of useful links.
www.blonz.com/nut.htm

Children's Nutrition Research Center, Baylor College of Medicine
Information on feeding kids the smart way.
www.bcm.tmc.edu/cnrc

iVillage
You can find out your personal daily calorie, fat, protein, and carbohydrate needs and much more by using the health calculators at this site.
www.ivillage.com/tools/healthcalc

Mayo Clinic Health Oasis
Click on Healthy Living Centers, then Food & Nutrition for tons of valuable information.
www.mayoclinic.com

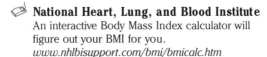

 178

National Heart, Lung, and Blood Institute
An interactive Body Mass Index calculator will
figure out your BMI for you.
www.nhlbisupport.com/bmi/bmicalc.htm

Nebraska Cooperative Extension
Reliable information about smart nutrition that's
easy to understand.
www.ianr.unl.edu/pubs/foods

Nutriquest
Cornell's Nutrition Q&A Service: Questions and
answers about nutrition from a reliable source.
www.nutrition.cornell.edu/nutriquest/nqhome.html

**NIDDK (National Institute of Diabetes and
Digestive and Kidney Diseases)
Weight Control Information Network**
A wealth of information on healthy eating and
weight loss.
www.niddk.nih.gov/health/nutrit/win.htm

**Sensible Nutrition Resource List for
Consumers**
A long list of references on nutrition, many of
them free or low cost.
www.nal.usda.gov/fnic/pubs/bibs/gen/98-senbl.htm

Tufts Nutrition Navigator
Rating guide to nutrition Web sites.
www.navigator.tufts.edu

 USDA Nutrient Database for Standard Reference
The mother of all calorie and fat-gram counters in a searchable format.
www.nal.usda.gov/fnic/cgi-bin/nut_search.pl

 Vegetarian Resource Group
Explore the vegetarian option at this informative site. *www.vrg.org*

Charts and Tables

Body Mass Index

If you want to figure out if you need to gain or lose weight, or if you weigh what you should for your height, the body mass index is considered by most experts to be the most reliable. A Body Mass Index Table can be found at
www.nhlbi.nih.gov/guidelines/obesity/bmi_tbl.htm

Find your height in inches across the top of the chart, then find your weight in pounds along the left side of it. The number where the two meet corresponds to your body mass. If it is:

- less than 18, you are underweight
- 18–24, you are at a healthy weight
- 25–29, you are overweight
- 30–40, you are obese
- more than 40, you are severely obese

This table applies to the average, healthy person of normal weight. You may or may not be some or all of these. Use it to get a general idea of how much fat you can safely eat, but take a closer look at how many calories you should be eating to achieve and maintain a weight that is healthy for you, and talk with a doctor to find out if your fat intake should be lower than 30 percent of total calories.

Recommended Fat Intake

(by age, gender, and weight)

Age	Weight in pounds	Daily fat intake by calories/gram 10%	20%	30%
Infants				
to 6 months	13	65/7	130/14.5	195/21.5
6–12 months	20	85/9.5	170/19	255/28.5
Children				
1–3 years	29	130/14.5	260/29	390/43.5
4–6 years	44	180/20	360/40	540/60
7–10 years	52	200/22	400/45	600/66.5
Teens, Females				
11–14 years	101	220/24.5	440/49	660/73.5
15–18 years	120	220/24.5	440/49	660/73.5
Teens, Males				
11–14 years	99	250/28	500/55.5	750/83.5
15–18 years	145	300/33.5	600/66.5	900/100

Recommended Fat Intake (continued)
(by age, gender, and weight)

Age	Weight in pounds	Daily fat intake by calories/gram		
		10%	20%	30%
Adults, Females				
19–24 years	128	220/24.5	440/49	660/73.5
25–50 years	138	220/24.5	440/49	660/73.5
51+ years	143	190/21	380/42	570/63.5
Adults, Males				
19–24 years	160	290/32	580/64.5	870/96.5
25–50 years	174	290/32	580/64.5	870/96.5
51+ years	170	230/25.5	460/51	690/76.5

Metric Conversion

These are approximate equivalents between metric units and those more commonly used in the United States.

Linear Measure (length, height)

1 centimeter = .4 inch

1 inch = 2.5 centimeters

1 meter = 40 inches

1 foot (12 inches) = .3 meter

1 yard (3 feet) = .9 meter

Volume (liquid)

1 ounce = 30 milliliters

1 cup = .25 liter

1 liter = 1 quart

1 gallon = 3.8 liters

Weight

1 microgram (mcg) = 1/1,000,000 gram

1 milligram (mg) = 1/1000 gram

1 gram = .035 ounce

1 ounce = 28 grams

1 kilogram = 2.2 pounds

1 pound = 453 grams

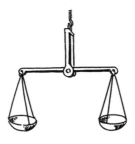

Glossary

amino acid—One of 80 naturally occurring complex molecules from which proteins are made; 20 are needed for human growth and metabolism; nine of these are considered "essential," because the body cannot manufacture them so they must be obtained from food; often called the "building blocks" of life.

antioxidant—a compound that interferes with the bonding of oxygen atoms; in the human body, oxidation is associated with some disease processes, and antioxidants are thought to inhibit those processes; some vitamins and vitamin precursors (beta-carotene and vitamins C and E) have antioxidant properties.

atherosclerosis—narrowing of the arteries as a result of deposition of fatty plaques; contributes to high blood pressure and heart disease and increases the risk of heart attack and stroke.

beta-carotene—an orange pigment that is a precursor of vitamin A; acts as an antioxidant (see also); found in bright yellow, orange, and leafy green vegetables and fruits.

carbohydrate—a carbon-hydrogen molecule that, as food, is the body's principal source of energy; one of the three major nutrients; edible carbohydrates can be simple (sugars), complex (starches), or very complex (fiber or cellulose); one gram of carbohydrate supplies four calories.

cholesterol—a waxy lipid manufactured by the liver or obtained through food, principally animal products; performs many vital functions in the body but represents a significant health risk when present at levels in excess of need.

complex carbohydrate—see *carbohydrate*

essential—Any nutritional component that must be obtained from food because the body cannot manufacture it; certain amino acids, fatty acids, vitamins, and minerals are termed "essential."

fat—a member of a family of chemical compounds called lipids; molecules that cannot be dissolved in water; found in many plants and animals, which use them as storehouses of energy; performs many vital functions in the human body; one of the three major nutrients; dietary fat can have a variety of molecular structures, which are termed saturated or unsaturated (monounsaturated and polyunsaturated), depending on the number of hydrogen atoms they contain; one gram of fat supplies nine calories.

fat-soluble—characteristic of vitamins and other substances that can be dissolved in fat or oil.

FDA—the U.S. Food and Drug Administration, the federal agency that regulates food, drugs, cosmetics, and medical devices.

fiber—a highly complex carbohydrate found in foods of plant origin that cannot be metabolized by humans;

although it supplies no calories, has numerous beneficial health effects; also called cellulose and roughage.

HDL—high density lipoprotein; a complex fat-protein molecule that transports *cholesterol* (see also) in the blood; called the "good" cholesterol, HDL does not contribute to atherosclerosis (see also); high levels of HDL are associated with a lower risk cardiovascular disease; see also *LDL*.

hydrogenation—a manufacturing process through which hydrogen atoms are added to *unsaturated fats* (see also) to make them taste and behave more like saturated fats; the process by which *trans fats* (see also) are produced.

LDL—low density lipoprotein; a complex fat-protein molecule that transports *cholesterol* (see also) in the blood; called the "bad" cholesterol, LDL is linked with *atherosclerosis* (see also); high levels of LDL are associated with a high risk cardiovascular disease; see also *HDL*.

lipid—a fat or fatlike substance.

lipoprotein—a combination molecule made up of lipid and protein, which transports cholesterol (see also) throughout the body in the blood; can be high or low density; see also *HDL* and *LDL*.

metabolism—the many chemical processes through which the body digests, uses, stores, and eliminates food and other substances to maintain life.

micronutrient—a nutritional substance needed by the body in minute amounts; vitamins and minerals are the principal micronutrients.

mineral—a nonorganic compound needed by the body for a wide range of metabolic processes.

monounsaturated—see *fat*.

omega-3—an essential fatty acid in the form of polyunsaturated fat that contributes to normal nervous system development and plays an important part in metabolism and hormone activity; thought to lower the level of triglycerides in the blood and also reduce the likelihood of blood clots; found in fatty fish, nuts, seeds, wheat germ, among other foods, and in breast milk.

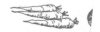

omega-6—an essential fatty acid in the form of polyunsaturated fat; found in soybean, corn, and safflower oils, egg yolks, organ meats, and other animal products; see also *omega-3*.

polyunsaturated—see *fat*

protein—a molecule made of *amino acids* (see also) that is found in animal products and, to a lesser degree, some foods of plant origin; one of the three major nutrients; as food, protein supplies four calories per gram; used by the body to make and maintain many tissues, including muscle; a secondary source of energy.

saturated—see *fat*

simple carbohydrate—see *carbohydrate*

trans fat—a fat manufactured by adding hydrogen atoms to unsaturated fat; associated with health risks including high cholesterol levels and atherosclerosis; see also *fat*.

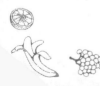

triglyceride—a lipid carried in the blood by very low-density lipoproteins (VLDL); high levels are associated with cardiovascular disease and diabetes.

USDA—United States Department of Agriculture, the federal agency that issues nutritional guidelines, provides information and educational material on food and nutrition issues, and maintains a database of the nutritional components of foods.

vitamin—an organic micronutrient needed by the body to support or perform many metabolic processes.

VLDL—very low-density lipoprotein; a combination molecule consisting of lipid and protein, which transports triglycerides through the blood.

water-soluble—characteristic of vitamins, minerals, or other substances that can be dissolved in water.

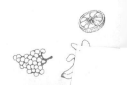